Understanding and Living Well With Post-Concussion Syndrome

Understanding and Living Well With Post-Concussion Syndrome

DR PRIYANKA PRADHAN & ANNA LEGGETT

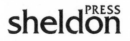

First published by Sheldon Press in 2022
An imprint of John Murray Press
A division of Hodder & Stoughton Ltd,
An Hachette UK company

1

This book is for information or educational purposes only and is not
intended to act as a substitute for medical advice or treatment. Any
person with a condition requiring medical attention should consult a
qualified medical practitioner or suitable therapist.

A CIP catalogue record for this title is available from the British Library

Trade Paperback ISBN 978 1 529 34614 5
eBook ISBN 978 1 529 34615 2

Typeset by KnowledgeWorks Global Ltd.

Printed and bound in Great Britain by Clays Ltd, Elcograf S.p.A.

John Murray Press policy is to use papers that are natural, renewable and
recyclable products and made from wood grown in sustainable forests.
The logging and manufacturing processes are expected to conform to the
environmental regulations of the country of origin.

John Murray Press
Carmelite House
50 Victoria Embankment
London EC4Y 0DZ

www.sheldonpress.co.uk

Priyanka:
To my husband and two amazing children, your love and support through this project have been unwavering, and I can't thank you enough.
To my parents, who taught me the importance of caring and inspired me to follow my heart and career path.

Anna:
This book is dedicated to my husband, Alex, and my three children, Danny, Kezzy and Chloe. You are my rocks. Thank you for everything.
I also wish to dedicate this book to all those people who've suffered a 'mild' brain injury but have experienced this invisible injury as anything but and have struggled to be understood and find a path towards recovery. You are brave beyond belief.

Acknowledgements

Priyanka

I would like to thank all my patients and clients who have trusted me enough to listen to their experiences and stories. I will always be humbled by the fact you have allowed me to assist you on your recovery journey in a collaborative and authentic way.

To my colleagues who have inspired and supported me to speak out for what I believe in professionally and politically, as well as be the voice for those that are yet to be heard. You know who you are.

To Anna Leggett, thank you for all your amazing work, time and dedication on this project. Your insight, compassion and knowledge shine through in a way that can only happen when someone has a lived experience of this condition and the multi-faceted challenges it brings.

Anna

I would like to thank the following people for the part they have played in my concussion recovery, in inspiring me and in me writing this book.

The publishing team at Sheldon Press, including Commissioning Editor Victoria Roddam, Meaghan Lim, Viv Church and Jenny Campbell for believing in this book and getting it published, encouraging and keeping me on track and providing your publishing expertise.

My dear husband, Alex, who has shown me much love and care and supported me in every possible way with my recovery. My three children, Danny, Kezzy and Chloe, who have shown love to me throughout and who have been so brave and resilient in the face of difficult times. The four of you are all my biggest cheerleaders and my main motivation for recovery.

My friends who stood by me and have been there for me, even though at times I haven't been the easiest person to be around or to understand. With special thanks to Alison, Clare, Janet, Julie, Julie B, Justine, Helen and William, Kirstie, Leonie, Michelle, Lucy, Rhonda and Sharon. You have no idea how much your friendship and support have meant to me, especially during those very difficult early weeks, months and years.

All the people who rallied round me in the early weeks and months and helped me with cleaning, shopping, childcare, ironing, laundry, taxi services, looking after our rabbits and moral support.

Kesgrave Scout Group (especially Cub leader Lesley Creasey and her husband John and Scout leaders Alan and Celia Comber) who have given tremendous support to us as a family and who have provided a safe, fun environment for my children, especially when I was struggling to look after them.

The Co-op Juniors Theatre Company, who have provided so much joy and encouragement to my two daughters and who've been accepting and supportive of me and our family situation. I'm grateful to the staff, parents and children. Thank you for providing this fun, creative outlet to my girls when life hasn't been the easiest for them.

All the many people who've experienced a concussion or more serious brain injuries who I've interacted with online in Facebook groups, on Instagram and Twitter. Thank you for sharing your tips, experiences, encouragement and support. I wish every one of you the best recovery possible. I'd especially like to thank David Bottomley of Post-Concussion Syndrome and mTBI Awareness Worldwide, GB Paraclimber Dave Bowes, Liz Meddings, founder of the UK Post-Concussion Syndrome Support Facebook group, Anne Johnston of Finding My Sparkle, Emma, Ellen, Esther and Karen.

Headway, the brain injury charity, my first source of information regarding concussion, and the members of staff on the helpline I spoke to.

The team at Headway Suffolk, including CEO Helen Fairweather, counsellor Julie Wilman, David Crane and Sophie Wellum-Mayes, and brainy dogs Bee and the late Hope. Thank you for your assistance and support and for the amazing six-week Understanding Brain Injury course that Alex and I attended and benefitted from.

My legal team who acted for me. I would not be where I am today without your help.

Dr Priyanka Pradhan, for your encouragement, expertise, support and wisdom and for the crucial role you played in my recovery. Thank you also for giving me the opportunity to co-author this book.

My GP, Dr John Lynch, who helped me to explore and access different healing options, including holistic ones.

Fiona Cole Goodwin, my kind friend and physiotherapist, who treated me at home when I couldn't get out and when I was at my worst. Thank you for your expertise in acupuncture and physiotherapy, friendship, listening skills, prayers and wisdom.

Felix Cory-Wright at Tollgate Healthcare, for your expertise in acupuncture and osteopathy, for teaching me the foundations of good health, and for helping me improve my mobility.

Lee Johnson, pain recovery coach, who helped me understand and manage chronic pain.

Peter Appel, embodiment and somatic expert, for your Movingness course and sharing your wisdom on all things equilibrium and movement.

Miriam Gauci Bongiovanni, coach and MindBody practitioner specializing in chronic pain and founder of Pain Outside the Box, for coaching me through a chronic pain flare up.

Justine Fawcett, neuro-occupational therapist, who helped me implement life strategies such as energy management, household organization and sleep hygiene.

The various health professionals I saw who advised, diagnosed, helped or treated me.

The inspiring people – health professionals, other professionals, concussion awareness campaigners, bloggers, writers and survivors of concussions and more serious brain injuries – who I've come across on my recovery journey, online or in person, who've helped countless people with their concussion and brain injury recoveries and who share their knowledge in this field with others. A mention here goes to Lynne Becker, founder of Power of Patients; trauma psychologist Dr James Zender; concussion survivor and functional neurologist Dr Titus Chiu; concussion survivor and founder of Faces of TBI Amy Zellmer; brain injury survivors and bloggers Michelle Munt, Brooke Trotter and Debbie Hampton; brain injury survivor, author and campaigner Cavin Balaster; brain injury survivor, author and founder of the Crash Support Network Dawne McKay; founder of Complete Concussion Management Dr Cameron Marshall; concussion survivor, author and course creator Ethan O'Brien; concussion survivor and personal trainer Brenda Shaughnessy; and brain injury survivor, author and motivational speaker Mark Kennedy. There are many more I haven't mentioned.

I'd like to thank Ajit Nawalkha, founder of Evercoach, and Dr Neeta Bhushan for inspiring me to study life coaching. Thank you, also, to members of the Evercoach community for encouraging me during the first year of my coaching journey.

Contents

Disclaimers

Priyanka: The information contained within this book is not meant to replace medical and neurological advice and treatment. It can be used as a tool to empower people with ongoing symptoms after a head injury, to seek ways to live the best life possible despite the day-to-day issues some people continue to experience.

Anna: I'm not a medical expert and my section of the book isn't a substitute for medical treatment and advice. Think of it as a guide to concussion recovery from someone who has walked the path before you. I share some of the different treatment options available as well as tools and strategies you can use straight away. This book is best used alongside the help you receive from your healthcare providers. Do discuss with them anything you have questions about or things that you think you might like to try. If you're still searching for specialist healthcare or if you're looking for some extra actions you can take between appointments, then this book will provide some pointers. There's an extensive reading and resources list at the end of this book, which provides many next steps and different avenues to explore to help you with your recovery.

About the authors

Priyanka

Dr Priyanka Pradhan is a Consultant Clinical Neuropsychologist with over 20 years' experience in the field of neurology and physical health. She has played a key role in developing neuropsychology services in the NHS and independent sector, with her main areas of specialism being movement and neuro-degenerative disorders, such as Parkinson's disease, along with traumatic brain injury and stroke. During her career, she has worked in various settings including maximum security hospitals, tertiary specialist hospitals and community services. She is on the British Psychological Society's (BPS) Specialist Register for Neuropsychologists, is Health and Care Professions Council registered and is the founder of Neurolistics Ltd. Her clinical practice is based in the UK.

As well as specialist neuropsychological diagnostic assessments, Dr Pradhan provides neuropsychological treatment packages for individuals, couples and groups living with neurological conditions. Dr Pradhan uses a variety of therapeutic approaches including Cognitive Behavioural Therapy (CBT), Acceptance and Commitment Therapy (ACT), Empowerment Behavioural Management Approach (EBMA), Motivational Interviewing and Compassionate Focused Therapy (CFT). Furthermore, Dr Pradhan is a qualified yoga teacher and has undertaken further training in the use of yoga practices and techniques alongside western trauma-focused practices to assist people in their recovery and growth. She also co-runs successful holistic retreats and continual professional development (CPD) events for colleagues working in neurorehabilitation.

For the past four years, Dr Pradhan has been a trustee on a board for a dynamic theatre company based in the Northwest of

England which is passionate about making theatre with young artists from backgrounds that are working-class and culturally diverse. She is also the chair on a board of an enterprise that provides accessible and targeted yoga classes for people living with a wide range of mental and physical health conditions. Dr Pradhan is currently training in Biodynamic Craniosacral Therapy (BCST) via Body College. She sees this as another avenue of treatment to assist her clients towards optimal health and well-being via the connection with and wisdom of their bodies.

Dr Pradhan's clinical approach is to draw upon all aspects of the individual, including their physical, emotional, cognitive, systemic, social and cultural status along with cutting-edge neuroscience research to provide truly bespoke interventions that encapsulate the mind, brain, body and spirit.

Anna

Anna Leggett is a wife and full-time mother of three children. She has worked in publishing, sales and administration and is part-trained as a counsellor. She experienced a mild head injury in a car accident in November 2016 and has been on a recovery journey ever since. More recently she has written blog posts on the subjects of concussion recovery and holistic living and undertaken training as a life coach. She lives in the Suffolk countryside and enjoys cooking, reading, swimming and walking.

Introduction

Priyanka

This book is drawn from my 20 years of clinical knowledge and experience of working in the field of neuropsychology. While the first part of my career was focused on neuropsychological diagnostics, increasingly over the years I have provided more psychological therapy and neurorehabilitation intervention to people and families living with long-term neurological conditions. In the last eight years, my work has been more focused on working with people who have ongoing symptoms following an injury to their head.

One of the people I have worked with is Anna, who has contributed significantly to this book by sharing her first-hand experience of what it's like to have a head injury and live with post-concussion syndrome (PCS). She details how she navigated through the health system and what tips and tools she has found to be beneficial. This is a book to share knowledge and fundamentally help people who like Anna may find themselves lost in a system that is not fit for purpose when it comes to this type of injury.

The book is for the small but significant percentage of people that continue to experience symptoms after having an injury to their head and so may get diagnosed with PCS. It is also aimed at their loved ones, as well as their GPs (given it can be challenging to understand the symptoms), to be better equipped to provide a treatment pathway for people with ongoing difficulties.

The book raises discussion points about how we describe and classify this injury, as well as the name we give it. There is a range of views and levels of understanding in the medical field which can on occasion be conflicting. From my clinical experience this can mean that people are told different things by different doctors and allied professionals about their diagnosis and prognosis. Understandably this can be confusing, frustrating and disheartening for individuals. It is not the purpose of this book to discuss the debates that surround head injury in the medical and legal world; instead, this book is to assist people on a challenging journey. It is my view that this is a complex injury that has to be understood on a multi-factorial level.

In terms of how people choose to use this book, while it is written in a way that will take you on a journey from understanding the relevant neuroscience to looking at ways to help you deal with ongoing symptoms and where to seek help, it can also be used as a reference to dip in and out of as required.

Anna

In November 2016, a 4 × 4 vehicle crashed into the back of my car while I was stationary in traffic at a roundabout near my hometown in Suffolk, UK. I sustained a concussion and musculoskeletal injuries to my head, neck, shoulder and back from the force of the impact. I was later diagnosed with post-concussion syndrome. My 3-year-old daughter was also in the car and sustained a concussion. However, for simplicity, this book is only about my own experiences.

Due to my injuries, I experienced a wide range of symptoms, including headaches, dizziness, vertigo, brain fog, light and sound sensitivity, cognitive and memory problems, fatigue, word finding difficulties and chronic pain.

My experience turned my life upside down. I couldn't drive and I frequently had to sleep for a couple of hours during the day and sometimes longer. It was difficult to walk, cook, organize myself, go out to busy places, read, write, look at a screen and use the computer. It was hard to be the mum and wife I wanted to be; my relationships with some family members and friends were affected; we ran into debt and I felt like I had aged 40 years overnight.

This was especially frustrating for me as some years before the accident I'd worked as an executive PA and a freelance copyeditor and I'd partially trained as a counsellor. At the time of the accident, I was a busy full-time mum to three children under nine years old. I'd previously been active, efficient and organized but now I was anything but.

There were many times when I thought I'd never get better. I often found myself thinking, 'Is my brain damaged forever?', 'Is this as good as it gets?', 'Will I ever be able to have a quality of life that I can feel happy about?'

Unfortunately, there wasn't a clear recovery pathway for me with the diagnosis of post-concussion syndrome. I experienced what many people with PCS go through: a long and challenging journey to understand my condition and find the right medical treatment for it.

I set about trying to figure out what I could do to improve and get better. I spent hundreds, if not thousands, of hours researching and trying to put together the pieces of the recovery jigsaw puzzle. It was a long and arduous journey of healing with many dead ends and frustrations. Thankfully, my very patient and long-suffering husband, my children and a number of caring friends provided much-appreciated encouragement, love and support during this time.

I trawled the internet and books for information on concussion recovery and pain relief. I struggled to read properly as the words would jump around in front of my eyes and I couldn't tolerate being on a screen for very long. My attention span and my ability to retain information were abysmal. But I persisted. I was obsessive about my quest to recover and I became fascinated with the brain and the nervous system. I just had to get better: the idea of staying this way was just too awful to contemplate.

Thankfully, I was gradually able to find the help of good healthcare providers; gain the assistance of a great specialist personal injury legal firm with access to medical experts; find help via the website and helpline of Headway, the UK brain injury charity, and my local Headway group and some online concussion recovery groups. They all provided many answers, solutions and much needed support. At the same time, I experimented with various supplements, nutritional plans, exercises, treatments and therapies. I was able to build up my exercise, stamina, reading, writing and many everyday skills. I embraced a wide range of lifestyle changes, natural modalities and mindset shifts. I was desperate, determined and driven.

Over the last few years, I've made good progress in my recovery. I still have a few struggles: mainly fatigue, some challenges with cognition, emotional regulation and pain, and I still find large social gatherings quite overwhelming. I do have to pace myself and sometimes I experience setbacks and flare-ups of symptoms. But I've come a long way from where I was and my life is, for the most part, pretty normal. I continue to put into practice many of the recommendations in this book. I keep seeing improvements, and at the same time I hold out hope for further healing.

I told myself that if I ever made a good enough recovery, I'd share my knowledge with others in a similar position. I never wanted anyone else to go through what I experienced: being met with blank looks; being misdiagnosed and not knowing what to do to get better.

I'm delighted to have the opportunity to co-author this book with Dr Priyanka Pradhan who started working with me in her capacity as a neuropsychologist around a year after my injury and supported me as I got back on my feet and rebuilt my life after my injury. Writing this book is a dream come true for me. For a long time after my accident, the physical and cognitive demands of writing were great and I could never have imagined undertaking such a project. As it turns out, writing has been cathartic and it has been an important part of my therapy. I've worked up to this by journaling, writing regular guest blog posts on concussion recovery and posting regularly on the topic on social media. I've also spent a year training part-time as a life coach, which I've loved.

PART ONE

1

Injury, the brain and the nervous system

The term concussion comes with varied understanding of its meaning within the medical world and among the general public.

There are a number of definitions of concussion, but on the whole it is described as an injury to the head or body that impacts on the function of the brain. Some definitions describe it as the most common and least serious type of traumatic brain injury (TBI). In the past it was assumed that someone would have to lose consciousness for a diagnosis of concussion to be made, but this is no longer the case.

The injury

While concussions usually occur when there has been a blow to the head, they can also be caused by the head being shaken or via an injury that causes a force to be transmitted through the body and brain (such as what happens to soldiers when they are near an explosion – this is called a blast injury).

There are many ways that injuries to the head can occur, and I have listed a few examples below:

- road traffic accidents involving all type of vehicles
- any sport, but especially those where there is a high risk of bangs to the head (e.g. boxing, rugby, football, ice hockey)
- falls, slips
- items falling on your head
- whiplash – the head is subjected to acceleration and deceleration forces without there being a direct knock or a bang to the head
- blast injuries.

When the head is knocked or subjected to forces that cause a jolt, the function of the brain can be impacted, as the brain is subject to a type of movement called 'acceleration and deceleration' (moving forwards and backwards at speed). It may also be affected by rotational forces, where the head and brain within the head are moved rapidly along other planes of direction (i.e. not just forwards or backwards).

As the brain is made of soft tissue suspended in cerebrospinal fluid within the skull, if the head is knocked or subjected to rapid external forces, the brain within the skull moves with a slight time delay. Movements in this time delay can cause a stretch of the nerves and blood vessels of the brain. This damage can then cause chemical and metabolic changes within the brain cells as well as bruising (indicating loss of blood), which affects how the brain cells function and communicate with each other.

Furthermore, a force to the head can cause a type of injury called a 'coup contrecoup' which affects not only the side of the brain where the skull was hit but also the opposite side of the brain. This happens as the brain is shifted by the forces on one side to the other. I have seen cases where someone has banged the back of their head but an injury occurred to the front of the brain, or cases where they had an impact on the left side of their head and suffered an injury on that side as well as the right side.

Any knock to the head can cause the brain's function to be temporarily halted or disrupted, which can result in a range of symptoms. If you have ever had a concussion, your vision may have been disturbed, you may have felt dizzy and become sensitive to noise and/or light, and you may have vomited, experienced a headache and felt confused. You may have also had emotional reactions like shock, anger, embarrassment or even shame.

Box 1. A brief summary of what happened when Anna suffered her injury

It was around 5 p.m. on a winter's evening in 2016. Anna was on her way home from dropping off her older children at her parents' home. Her youngest daughter, who was three at the time, was in her child safety seat in the back of the car. She was in rush hour traffic and recalls waiting for about 10–15 minutes in stationary traffic near a roundabout on an A road. Anna had the handbrake on and was listening to a CD. She describes experiencing a 'violent jolt out of the blue'. She did not realize what had happened and even thought it could have been an explosion. Anna felt her head jolt forwards and then backwards, hitting the headrest. This was clear in her mind as it happened so quickly. Anna describes feeling a sensation in her head and right eye socket as her head was thrust forward and also felt a jolt in her torso. She had her seat belt on. Anna then realized that her car must have been hit and rang 999. The phone operator asked if anyone had been hurt and because Anna said no, they informed her that the police would not be dispatched. Anna saw a lay-by to the left, so she pulled over and got out of her car. She recalls it being pitch black, and also feeling embarrassed. As she walked to the back of her car she recalls the driver of the other car, a man, walking over and apologizing. Her memory from this point onwards gets somewhat patchy.

Anna does recall experiencing some confusion over swapping details: she remembers walking off before she had given the man her details, and he had to call her back. She feels that she was not really 'with it' and had an urge to get home. The other driver took photos of the damage to the cars on his phone.

Anna's memory got more vague and patchy. She does not recall the route she took to get home nor getting out of the car when she arrived home. She also does not recall what she did that night, though she knows that her husband cooked their evening meal. She recalls becoming cold and shivery later on in the evening. Anna also describes a sense of 'zoning out', feeling very tired and incapable of doing anything.

The brain

Before I go any further, I think it would be useful to give you an overview of the brain and the nervous system.

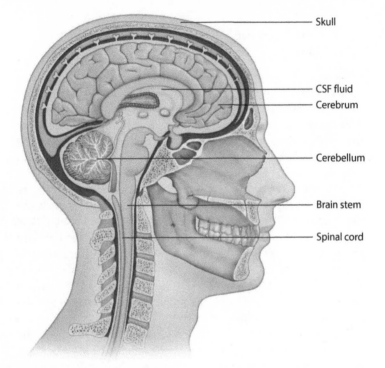

Skull

CSF fluid
Cerebrum

Cerebellum

Brain stem

Spinal cord

Cross-section diagram showing elements of the central nervous system, including the brain.

The brain is encased in a strong outer shell of bone – our skull. Like many bones in the body, it is there to protect delicate inner organs and tissues and provide a frame or structure. The brain is made of soft tissue that is cushioned by spinal fluid within the skull.

The brain gets more complex in function from the bottom to the top and back to front. The brain stem, at the bottom, which is the link to your spinal cord, is responsible for basic but fundamental bodily functions such as breathing regulation, heart rate and temperature. These are also known as 'autonomic functions'. This is the first part of the nervous system to develop in the embryo. Moving up, we have the cerebellum, which is responsible for abilities such as balance and coordination. Then we have the cerebrum, the largest part of the brain, divided into two halves called hemispheres, which are then further divided into four sections called lobes. Each lobe is associated with different cognitive, emotional and behavioural functions, which are detailed below:

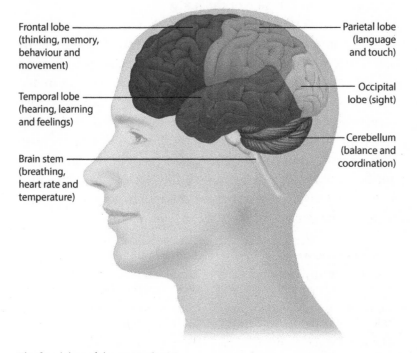

Frontal lobe
(thinking, memory,
behaviour and
movement)

Temporal lobe
(hearing, learning
and feelings)

Brain stem
(breathing,
heart rate and
temperature)

Parietal lobe
(language
and touch)

Occipital
lobe (sight)

Cerebellum
(balance and
coordination)

The four lobes of the cortex (brain).

The red is the front and top part of the brain, and the orange part is the back and bottom. The two hemispheres mirror each other, so each side (left and right) has a frontal, parietal, temporal and occipital lobe.

The left side of the brain is associated with memory for verbal material (e.g. stories, names, words) and language skills. The right side of the brain is associated with memory for non-verbal material (faces, pictures, diagrams) and visual perceptual skills. In the field of neurology, we refer to the left side of the brain as the 'dominant hemisphere' because this is where language is located in humans during normal development. It is important to note that the brain connects to the body in a contralateral way: the left side of the brain controls the right side of the body, and the right side of the brain affects the left side of the body.

When someone has what we call a 'focal injury' on one side of their brain, such as a stroke, it can affect the function of the opposite side of their body. For example, if the stroke occurs on the left side of the brain, the person's ability to speak or understand the speech of others is usually affected, and they have weakness or paralysis in parts of the right side of their body. Those that have strokes that occur on the right side of the brain tend to have more visual-perceptual issues which can involve not being able to pay attention to the left side of their visual field (called visual neglect) and have loss of sensation and/or power in the left side of their body.

Left hemisphere	Right hemisphere
Receives sensory input from the *right* side of the body	Receives sensory input from the *left* side of the body
Controls the muscles on the *right* side of the body	Controls the muscles on the *left* side of the body
Memory for verbal information, i.e. words, letters, numbers	Memory for visual information, i.e. faces, places, objects
Language functions, i.e. verbal output and understanding others' speech	Visual, spatial and perceptual skills
Mathematical and analytical skills	Rhythm and music
Logic and linear thinking	Holistic thinking
Time and sequencing	Intuition and imagination

As well as the brain being divided into four lobes (frontal, parietal, temporal and occipital), the main part of the brain (also known as the cerebrum) is divided into 'grey' (cortex or neocortex) and 'white' (subcortex) regions.

The cortex is the outer layer of the brain. It is about 3mm thick but highly folded, creating a massive surface area that contains billions of neurons. Only mammals have a cortex and for humans, the cortex is where many of the higher-level cognitive functions take place (e.g. rational decision making, planning, calculation and language).

The subcortex, which means 'beneath the cortex', is where we process more primitive functions (e.g. emotional reactions). However, cortical and subcortical areas are continually interacting (e.g. deciding when to suppress anger).

A brief outline of the key subcortical structures and their functions is detailed below:

Corpus callosum: relays information between the two hemispheres

Hypothalamus: regulates the endocrine system, the immune system and the autonomic nervous system (which is why all these three systems are connected)

Amygdala: emotional centre

Pituitary: the master gland

Thalamus: relays information between the cortex and the subcortex

Hippocampus: learning and memory

Fornix: cognition and episodic memory recall

Cerebellum: movement

Brain stem: relays information from the body, governs vital functions.

The limbic system comprises a few of these subcortical structures and its main function is to facilitate memory storage and retrieval, establish emotional states and provide a link between the functions of the cortex (grey matter) with the unconscious, autonomic functions of the brain stem. While the sensory cortex, motor cortex and associated areas allow you to perform tasks, the limbic system helps motivate you to do those tasks.

While the brain is divided into sections and there is what we call 'localization and lateralization of function', the brain works in sync and sends messages within the different lobes and regions in order to process information and execute responses. A major structure of importance in helping the two hemispheres integrate information is the corpus callosum, a white matter structure consisting of several nerve tracts that connect the two halves of the hemispheres. This allows the hemispheres to process motor, sensory and cognitive signals in unison and communicate back and forth, which harmonizes the intricate functions of the brain.

The corpus callosum also plays a crucial role in eye movement and vision by connecting both halves of the hemispheres of the visual field. This white matter nerve bundle allows us to see and then identify objects by connecting the visual cortex in brain language centres (i.e. our vision helps us see it, but our language and memory help us name/identify it). Also, the corpus callosum processes tactile information in the parietal lobes and transmits between the brain hemispheres to help us identify touch and space. It helps to maintain the balance of attention and awareness and so plays a vital overall role in cognition.

Here are two views of the brain. The first is the cross-section from a side-on view, while the second shows the brain if looking at it from the front.

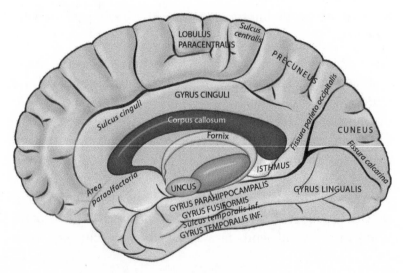

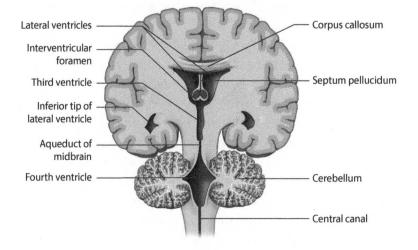

Lateral ventricles

Interventricular foramen

Third ventricle

Inferior tip of lateral ventricle

Aqueduct of midbrain

Fourth ventricle

Corpus callosum

Septum pellucidum

Cerebellum

Central canal

When the integrity of the corpus callosum is damaged, it affects cognitive functioning. For example, while language comprehension occurs mainly in the left temporal lobe, in order to make a response verbally, we need to engage the left frontal part of the brain where verbal production is located.

Lastly, let's look at the cells of the brain, which are called neurons. Most neurons can be likened to trees. They have a cell body that is similar to a trunk of a tree, which then has fibres that extend out of it, similar to roots (axons) and branches (dendrites). The job, in fact the compulsion, of these axons and dendrites is to seek out such structures in other neurons in order to connect and communicate. They communicate by sending and receiving signals, which is fundamental for the brain and body to function. These connections are minimal at birth but increase as we grow via all the things we see, do and learn. All our experiences create a bigger network of connections in the brain, which leads to brain development.

Neurons communicate via a synapse, a tiny gap between the axon of one neuron and the dendrite of another, which serves as a contact point for messages to be transmitted between neurons. When neurons send or receive messages, they transmit electrical impulses along their axons, which results in a release of neuro-chemicals between the neurons. Most axons, which can vary in length, are covered in a myelin sheath that accelerates the transmission of electrical signals along the axon.

Neurons are a unique form of cell. For a long time, it was thought that they do not get replaced if they are damaged, but due to contemporary evidence around 'neuroplasticity', we know that existing neurons can change, grow and reorganize by making new connections between existing neurons. As such, we have learnt that the brain can change and adapt for our entire lives.

You may have also heard the brain referred to as being made up of 'grey and white matter'. The 'grey matter' is the area of the brain where the actual processing is done, referred to as grey because of the colour of the nuclei contained in the cells that make it up. The 'white matter' refers to those parts of the brain and spinal cord that are responsible for communication between the various grey matter regions and between the grey matter and the rest of the body. The white matter is so called because it contains many nerve fibres or neurons that are sheathed in the white fatty insulating protein called myelin. So, grey matter is the cortex and white matter is the subcortex. In essence, the grey matter is where the processing is undertaken and the white matter is the channel of communication.

The nervous system

The nervous system is a vast array of terminals that meander through the whole body and each part of the system plays a vital role in how information is experienced, communicated and responded to by the body and brain. It is divided into two main systems:

1 The central nervous system (CNS) (brain and spinal cord)
2 The peripheral nervous system (all nerves that travel to the body from the brain and vice versa).

Let's focus on the peripheral nervous system, which contains all the nerves that lie outside the central nervous system. The primary role of the peripheral nervous system is to connect and send information from the central nervous system to the organs, limbs and skin and vice versa so that we can respond to sensory information coming from our external and internal environment. These nerves extend from the central nervous system to the outermost areas of the body.

The peripheral nervous system functions are to:

- connect the central nervous system to the organs, limbs and skin
- carry sensory and motor information to and from the central nervous system
- allow the brain and spinal cord to receive and send information to other areas of the body
- regulate involuntary body functions like heartbeat and breathing.

The peripheral nervous system itself is divided into two parts: the somatic nervous system and the autonomic nervous system. Each of these components plays a critical role in how the peripheral nervous system operates.

The somatic system is the part of the peripheral nervous system responsible for carrying sensory and motor information to and from the central nervous system. The somatic nervous system derives its name from the Greek word 'soma', which means 'body'. It is also responsible for voluntary movement (picking up a cup, kicking a ball, stirring a spoon). This system contains two major types of neurons:

Motor neurons: Also called 'efferent' neurons, motor neurons carry information from the brain and spinal cord to muscle fibres throughout the body. These motor neurons allow us to take physical action in response to stimuli in the environment.

Sensory neurons: Also called 'afferent' neurons, sensory neurons carry information from the nerves to the central nervous system. It is these sensory neurons that allow us to take in sensory information and send it to the brain and spinal cord.

The autonomic nervous system (ANS) is the part of the peripheral nervous system that is responsible for regulating involuntary body functions, such as blood flow, heartbeat, digestion and breathing. These functions occur below our conscious awareness and essentially carry on in the background. We do not have to think about breathing, or making sure our heart is beating, or digesting our lunch. In other words, it is the autonomic system that controls aspects of the body that are usually not under voluntary control.

The autonomic system is further divided into two branches:

Sympathetic nervous system: By regulating the fight or flight response, the sympathetic system prepares the body to expend energy when necessary.

This branch evolved in relation to threat, predominantly in the environment of our ancestors. If information came through their senses of potential danger to their safety (hearing a rustling in the bush, smelling fire, seeing a dangerous animal in the distance), an alarm system went off in the brain. A cascade of nerve and hormone signals then released, triggering a response that prepares the body to either stay and fight or run as fast as possible to get away from immediate danger. This process has not really changed as we have evolved over millions of years, despite the significant reduction in many environmental threats.

When action is needed, the sympathetic system triggers the release of hormones including adrenaline and cortisol.

Adrenaline increases the heart and breathing rates, boosts energy supplies and blood flow to muscles, dilates pupils and activates sweat secretion. Cortisol (also known as the stress hormone) increases sugars (glucose) in the bloodstream, enhances the brain's use of glucose and increases the availa-bility of substances that repair tissues (in case we get hurt in battle). Cortisol also helps to curb functions that would be non-essential or even harmful in a fight or flight situation. As such, it plays a role in suppressing immune, digestive, reproduction and growth systems, as it sees this as a waste of energy during this time where survival is its main focus. Our cognitive functions also go into problem solving for survival purposes, becoming highly focused on the task in hand, while any thoughts relating to imagination, creativity or connective social interactions are put aside.

Parasympathetic nervous system: After a period of necessary sympathetic activation, the body and brain's stress response systems and hormone levels need to be able to return to 'normal', given that all the time a person is in sympathetic activation, bodily functions that are necessary for health, well-being and growth (immunity, digestion, reproduction and growth) are put on hold to conserve energy for survival. This is why sometimes this branch is referred to as the 'rest, digest and restore' system.

The parasympathetic system helps maintain normal body functions and conserve physical resources. Once a threat has passed, this system will slow the heart rate, slow breathing, reduce blood flow to muscles and constrict the pupils. This allows us to return our bodies to a normal resting state. This is also the place where we can be open to making social connec-tions, allow ourselves to think creatively and engage in playful endeavours. As we emerge from the zone of threat and danger, we can restore depleted resources used when in sympathetic activation.

Sympathetic branch of ANS	Parasympathetic branch of ANS
Pupils are dilated	Pupils are constricted
Saliva production is inhibited (dry mouth)	Saliva production is stimulated
Bronchi in the lungs are relaxed and heart rate is increased	Bronchi in the lungs are constricted and heart rate is decreased
Digestion is inhibited	Digestion is stimulated
Glucose release in the liver is stimulated	Gallbladder is stimulated
Adrenaline release is stimulated	Adrenaline production is inhibted
Bladder is relaxed	Bladder is contracted
Sexual climax, rectum is contracted	Rectum is relaxed

To understand the relationship between the SNS and the PSNS, we often use the analogy of a car and the different functions of the pedals. The SNS is analogous to the accelerator, dominant when we need to rouse the body systems (e.g. increase heart rate, direct more blood to the muscles) often, but not always in response to stress or danger – like the car speeding up to get us where we need to be. However, just as the car needs refuelling in order to keep going, the body needs to recoup and restore. In this way the PSNS acts as a brake pedal, helping to slow down the car and giving us time to rebuild resources. Also, if the car was always going at maximum speed, it would be more susceptible to damage, along with wear and tear. Equally, long-term activation of the SNS results in hyperarousal, which is fatiguing to the body and brain, and lowers immune system functioning, making the individual more susceptible to illness.

A healthy autonomic system has the two branches working in tandem, with the PSNS (rest, digest and restore) being the default and the SNS (fight, flight, freeze) ramping up and dampening its activity as and when required. However, when there has been significant trauma, the brain is on high alert for any other threats to existence. This threat can be physical, emotional or social, actual or perceived. As such, our understanding of the role of the autonomic nervous system and physiological state not only plays out in the health of our brain and body, but also in our social behaviour.

The Polyvagal Theory (PVT), which has come out of the pioneering work of Dr Stephen Porges, is fundamentally an updated theory about the ways in which the autonomic nervous system functions for human beings. It has shone a light on the importance of the vagus nerve. The vagus nerve, which is also known as the 'wandering nerve', has a left and a right branch that runs from the brain via the throat to the lungs, the heart, the stomach and then the intestines, and is the longest nerve of the ANS. The vagus nerve also communicates with an individual's immune system.

The premise of the theory (or some would say a working model of the autonomic nervous system) is that humans need safety – our biology is fiercely devoted to this – but this is in tandem with the biological drive for survival. PVT has three core principles which are co-regulation, neuroception and hierarchy.

Co-regulation refers to the ANS sending out and searching for cues of safety or danger. How do we balance between the drive to survive and the longing to connect, given that human beings are social creatures? While these two primary experiences can coexist, sometimes they work together, and other times they work in opposition to each other. Depending on our experiences in life, how we unconsciously interpret cues from other people will be affected. As such, while our nervous system is shaped and regulated by our interactions with others, it can also be triggered to be activated by others. For example, imagine you are invited to a party and you do not know who else will be going. As you enter the room, it is loud and crowded and you see a group of strangers huddled together, laughing. In this situation, you may unconsciously pick up cues of rejection and/or social threat. In a micro moment, your sympathetic nervous system leaps into action, signalling you to turn around and leave the party (flight), or perhaps head straight to the buffet and fill a plate to keep you occupied. Just then, you notice one of the guests breaking away from the crowd and walking towards you. She smiles and has an open, welcoming posture. Almost instantly, your breathing slows, your heart rate goes down and your body relaxes into the experience of *'Ah, I'm safe now'*. Your ANS has just guided you from a sympathetic state to a ventral vagal one, permitting what Porges calls your social engagement system to come fully online. You are now calm, ready to connect – and maybe able to initiate a new conversation.

These cues for safety and danger operate beneath our awareness. The three main elements of our autonomic nervous system – sympathetic, dorsal and ventral – act as our largely subconscious surveillance system, working in the background to read subtle signals of safety or threat. Dr Porges coined the term 'neuro-ception' to describe the way our ANS scans the environment and our internal world for cues of safety and danger without any assistance from our thinking brain. Rather, it is a visceral feeling that lets us know if we are safe or not in any given situation.

Safety comes when we feel connected within ourselves and with others. Here is a very brief and simplistic description of the two main pathways of the parasympathetic branch:

- **Ventral vagal:** responds to cues of safety and supports a sense of centredness and readiness for social engagement.
- **Dorsal vagal:** responds to cues of life-threat, causing shutdown, numbness and disconnect from others. Someone who dissociates has found refuge in the dorsal vagal state.

In terms of the hierarchy, the earliest evolutionary circuit was the dorsal vagal, where shutdown was the only option, then came the sympathetic response where we were mobilized to survive (i.e. flight or fight). The latest to develop was the ventral vagal circuit, which allows us to connect to the self, others and the world. It also allows us to be able to acknowledge our and others' distress without getting overwhelmed. It helps us be resourceful and to reach out for support when we can identify we need it but also recognize when others need support and offer it to them.

Ventral vagal	Social engagement system	Communication and connection – engagement with ourselves, others and the world. 'I feel connected and content'. Helps us rest/digest. Location where vagus nerve is stimulated most: face, throat, chest.
Sympathetic	Fight/flight	Mobilization – first line of defence. Utilisation of a body's resources to deal with a stessor/threat. 'I'm in danger. I need to fight or run away.' Increase of heart rate and muscle tension. Location where vagus nerve stimulated most: spinal cord.
Dorsal vagal	Shut down/ collapse/freeze	Immobilization – second line of defence when fight/flight is not possible. 'I can't cope. I need to shut down/cut off.' Bodily functions 'freeze' to preserve life. Location where vagus nerve stimulated most: diaphragm, gut, viscera.

When we have an autonomic nervous system that is regulated – that is, can respond to threat or danger when we need it to, but can rebalance to a state where our resources can be replenished and restored – it provides a platform for us to be able to interact with ourselves, others and the world in adaptative, connective and nourishing ways. This allows us to be in a healthy state rather than in a state of long-term survival mode, which can have a detrimental impact on physical, psychological and spiritual well-being.

So, what has all this got to do with having an injury to the head? Everything you have read here about the brain and nervous system is provided to help you understand a large proportion of your ongoing symptoms (or the symptoms of loved ones) and provides a foundation to learning about living well with post-concussion syndrome. In the next chapter, we will explore what exactly a concussion is, and what post-concussion syndrome is and how it is related to brain injury. I will also briefly touch upon and discuss the terminology and labels that are in use in the medical field.

2

Head injury: signs, symptoms and labels

What range of symptoms can people experience after a head injury, what do they mean and what do they tell us about what someone has experienced and/or suffered? During my time in clinical practice, I have gathered information from a large number of people of different ages and from all walks of life about the injuries they have experienced and how the symptoms may have evolved over time. While there are similarities, no one person's constellation or experience of symptoms is exactly the same. This is because an injury to the head can be so variable and we are all so unique that our biological and psychological responses to an injury can be wide ranging. In Chapter 3, we will look more in detail at potential vulnerability factors that may influence the degree to which a head injury affects someone. For this section, though, let's focus on the terminology and biology in relation to the symptoms.

The understanding you have or the diagnosis you have been given since your head injury or concussion will depend on the professionals you have seen along your journey. For many people who continue to have persistent symptoms after a head injury, a diagnosis may have been given of 'post-concussion syndrome' which is listed in The International Classification of Diseases, 10th revision (ICD-10), published by the World Health Organization (WHO). Or you could have a diagnosis of Postconcussional Disorder (PCD) which is listed in the Diagnostic and Statistical Manual of Mental Disorders (DSM-5) and is published by the American Psychiatric Association. The most recent consensus statement on concussion in sport defines a concussion as a

> TBI induced by biomechanical forces and caused by either a direct blow to the head, face, neck or elsewhere on the body with an impulsive force transmitted to the head, which typically results in the rapid onset of short-lived impairment of neurological function that resolves spontaneously, but in some cases, the signs and symptoms evolve over a number of minutes to hours. The acute clinical signs and symptoms reflect a functional disturbance rather than a structural injury and may or may not include loss of consciousness. Resolution of the clinical and cognitive features typically follows a sequential course. McCrory et al. (2017)

Some individuals may also have been given the diagnosis of mild traumatic brain injury (mTBI). Mild TBI is defined as a head injury associated with loss of consciousness of less than 30 minutes, Glasgow Coma Scale of 13 or higher, post-traumatic amnesia of less than 24 hours, altered level of awareness of less than 24 hours and normal neuroimaging. Let's explore what some eminent neurologists say with regards to these labels and diagnoses.

Two highly respected neurologists recently published a paper entitled 'Concussion is not a true diagnosis' (Smith & Stewart 2020). In this paper they detail how the term concussion is often used interchangeably with mTBI, but that there is nothing 'mild' about the condition for many individuals. They go on to say that the use of the term 'concussion' is no more sophisticated than the term 'consumption', the condition we have now come to know as Mycobacterium tuberculosis. As with 'consumption', concussion does not encompass the nature of the illness with regards to the underlying patho- logical process, as its focus is on the symptoms. However, there is increasing evidence that the symptoms people experience acutely (up to four weeks), sub-acutely (four weeks to a year) and chronically (one year onwards) reflect structural and physiological disruption of brain networks, particularly the vulnerable white matter predominantly found in the subcortical regions of the brain. The specific damage then results in 'diffuse axonal injury', a concept I will explain below. Another team of neurologists headed by Professor David Sharp also highlights the drawbacks of using the term concussion. In a paper entitled *'Concussion is confusing us all'*, the authors open with the sentence 'It is time to stop using the term concussion as it has no clear definition and no pathological meaning' (Sharp and Jenkins, 2015). They argue that using the term concussion is impacting on the management of individuals given this diagnosis. They note that historically the term concussion was used to describe those that were briefly and temporarily affected by a head injury but did not go on to suffer long-term sequelae. However, they highlight that:

> The symptoms of concussion are highly variable in duration and can persist for many years with no reliable predictors of outcome. Using vague terminology for post-traumatic problems leads to misconceptions and biases in the diagnostic process, producing uninterpretable science, poor clinical guidelines and confused policy. We propose that the term concussion should be avoided.

These authors propose that instead of using the term concussion, neurologists and healthcare professionals should classify the severity of the injury to the brain and then attempt to precisely diagnose the underlying cause of post-traumatic symptoms.

For many people, to have a diagnosis with the words 'traumatic brain injury', even if the descriptor 'mild' precedes it, can bring up an understandably negative emotional reaction. I have many clients who in fact prefer to use the term PCS when referring to their difficulties and what they are experiencing after an injury to their head. What is important to note here is that not every injury to the head causes a mild TBI and not every mild TBI results in persistent PCS. Given the nature of my work,

I tend to only see those that have ongoing issues, but there are thousands of people who recover within a matter of weeks after a head injury and/or concussion. From a clinical perspective, one factor that plays a part in the persistence of ongoing issues and outcomes is how people interact and respond to their symptoms. We will be looking at this in more detail in later chapters. My main goal when working with individuals who suffer this type of injury is to help them understand and find ways to overcome the day-to-day difficulties they have been experiencing since the injury, and to have a shared knowledge and understanding of what can assist adjustment and recovery for them.

There is a reticence among some clinicians to give the diagnosis of mTBI to someone who has had an injury to their head or neck but has ongoing symptoms. There are a number of reasons for this. Some clinicians argue that if you tell someone they have mTBI, then that person will start behaving as if they have a brain injury. They propose that these individuals will become hypervigilant to any changes in their functioning and attribute it to the brain injury. Some clinicians have the view that it is too traumatic to give a diagnosis with the term 'brain injury' as it suggests permanent damage with no hope for recovery. Some clinicians hold the position that the symptoms people experience that last beyond three months are psychologically manifested and are not due to pathophysiological changes in the brain, as the brain should have recovered by the three-month mark. However, we are learning from recent and robust research studies that this is an arbitrary time point.

There is also quite a range of opinions as to what PCS is in the UK versus North America. In the UK, being given a diagnosis of PCS can come (in some cases, not all) with negative connotations for the individual. Some professionals see the symptoms associated with PCS as more psychologically mediated as opposed to being the result of organic changes in the brain after neuro-trauma.

My own perspective on this is that if we do not fully and correctly understand the reason underlying the symptoms, it is hard to properly treat them.

There are many different systems that have been developed to classify the severity of a brain injury. The most commonly used one is the Mayo Clinic classification. It uses a number of indicators to which to compare the type of injury and symptoms someone may present with. These include the period of loss of consciousness, the degree of anterograde amnesia (loss of memory before the injury), post-traumatic amnesia (duration of loss of memory after the injury), Glasgow Coma Scale (GCS) score (a tool used to measure how much someone is responsive and conscious after an injury, scored out of 15), and the degree of injury that can be seen on a standard scan (e.g. bleeding in the brain, injury to the skull). The three classifications of brain injury severity on the Mayo classification are Moderate to Severe (definite), Mild (probable) and Symptomatic (possible).

While this classification of the severity of the brain injury is important for emergency treatment of life-threatening situations (e.g. a significant bleed on the brain), it doesn't help clinicians, or those with the injuries themselves, understand symptoms and injuries that are mild and/or symptomatic. It might even affect the type of care received – for example, someone with a 'mild' TBI might have persistent symptoms, yet treatment and support are withdrawn too soon, but someone with a 'severe' injury can have a more favourable outcome than generally expected.

The effects of trauma to the brain can be transient or persistent and as such, so can the symptoms. You may experience an injury to the head and have some immediate symptoms, such as confusion, feeling dazed, headache, light sensitivity and nausea/vomiting. Over the following few days and weeks these symptoms abate and you return to how you were pre-injury. Other people may experience these types of symptoms acutely (up to four weeks after the injury) and while some may resolve (e.g. vomiting), other symptoms may persist and further symptoms may appear. These might be physical symptoms (headaches, changes in sleep, pain, visual disturbance, issues with balance) or cognitive (poor memory, concentration and decision making) and neurobehavioural (irritability, anger, fatigue, anxiety, low mood). Symptoms can vary from individual to individual and can have a range of impacts on someone's day-to-day function, work capability and social pursuits.

There has been a lot of investigation into the potential reasons why some people go on to develop persistent symptoms after an injury to the head (be that contact or non-contact). A number of 'vulnerability factors' have been identified, including previous head trauma, having a history of psychological or psychiatric diagnosis, and being female. This will be discussed further in Chapter 3.

In some instances injury to the brain can be picked up on scans such as CT and MRI, and these standard tools are used to rule out anything imminently serious like major bleeding or structural damage that can be treated with surgical intervention. However, they are not sensitive enough to identify the microscopic changes that can occur after an injury to the head and brain. Even though MRI scanning is more detailed than a CT scan, often a standard MRI would be reported as 'normal' after someone has experienced an injury to their head. However, a negative MRI result does not mean there is no damage to the brain, albeit on a microscopic level.

Diffuse axonal injury (DAI) is the term used to refer to the damage caused when the head is subjected to acceleration/deceleration forces (see Chapter 1). The axons of the neurons (brain cells) get stretched and sometimes sheared due to the delayed movement of the brain within the skull when the head is moved at speed or is subjected to a force. Researchers have found that the deep midline structures in the brain, in particular the fornix, which is part of the limbic system, as well as the corpus callosum (which connects the two hemispheres of the brain), are most substantially affected, compared to the cortex (grey matter). Also, the white matter is more vulnerable to injury than grey matter because it becomes more brittle when it is rapidly stretched. This injury is less consistently associated with immediate concussion symptoms (like loss of consciousness) despite being associated with microscopic structural changes in the brain.

As we saw in Chapter 1, the main function of these white matter tracts is to relay messages and information between different parts of the brain. When they are ruptured, it takes more time and energy for information to pass between different areas of the brain, and cognitive dysfunction occurs predominantly in the domains of memory, executive function and processing speed. These cognitive functions are associated with frontal and subcortical regions of the brain, the areas most vulnerable to damage after this type of acceleration/deceleration injury.

Box 2. Anna's experience over the first few days following the car accident

After the accident, Anna contacted her insurance company, but initially got mixed up and contacted the company that holds her house insurance. Anna told me that she only recalled bits of information from the phone conversation, which is unlike her. It was during this conversation that she noticed that her right shoulder was sore, and that she felt very tired.

The next day Anna noticed the pain in her right shoulder had started to spread throughout her back and neck. Her memory continues to be patchy for that day; she recalls the man who hit her car calling and asking about the damage, but she could not recall all of the conversation. Anna also recalls that she contacted the general practitioner (GP) to make an appointment and that the replacement car arrived at her home, as the damage to her car meant it was not roadworthy. Anna recalls speaking to her mother to let her know what had happened and feeling relieved that her mother would drop her two elder children back as she did not feel up to driving. Anna's memory continued to have gaps for the next few days and the levels of pain in her upper body increased. Anna visited the out of hours GP and was advised to take Ibuprofen for her pain.

Over the next couple of days, Anna started to experience increased pain and feeling 'not quite right'. Anna carried on with her day-to-day activities and looking after her children, although her recall of the events was not as clear as it usually would have been. She also gave a number of examples of her not behaving and inter-acting with others as she usually did and finding it a struggle to have conversations with multiple people at the same time.

About four days after the accident, Anna noticed that her memory was not improving. She also started to feel dizzy, off balance and confused, as well as having some issues with her vision. Around the one-week mark after the accident, she saw her GP who diagnosed her with whiplash and concussion, and she was advised to self-refer to an NHS physiotherapy service. With regards to her visual problems, the GP responded that he'd never heard of a concussion causing vision problems and completed a brief eye test, which Anna passed. As such, he suggested that she probably needed a new glasses prescription and to make an appointment with her optician. Anna recalls leaving the GP's room but having to go back as she had forgotten to ask for painkillers for her neck, shoulder and back, which was one of the main reasons she had made the appointment.

What you may notice is that not all of Anna's symptoms showed up immediately but instead evolved over a number of days. She continued to participate in her daily life but found changes in her functioning compared to before the accident. Anna did not attend hospital or have any reason to think that her symptoms were due to microscopic injury due to her brain within her head being subjected to acceleration/deceleration forces when her car was hit from behind. However, later, Anna was diagnosed as having suffered a traumatic brain injury, specifically diffuse axonal injury, as well as whiplash and soft tissues injuries to her neck, shoulder and elbow, by a neurologist who examined her and took a detailed history regarding the nature, evolution and persistence of her symptoms since the accident. Anna was also diagnosed as having an audio-vestibular injury which will be detailed in Chapter 6.

With increased long-term prospective research studies being undertaken into the nature of symptoms people report following a head injury and the impact on their day-to-day lives, the notion that brain injury can be present only if it is visible on standard scanning (i.e. CT and MRI) and will improve after three months in all cases is slowly being refuted. One very large study followed people for around one year following their injury and compared those who had identifiable changes on brain scans with those who didn't and found no significant difference in the impact of the symptoms following head injury between the two groups (*TRACK TBI Study*, 2018).

A trajectory of increased cognitive, emotional and behavioural symptoms does not occur in every case of head injury. But many people (from 10 to 50 per cent) do continue to have symptoms after three months that are related to brain injury rather than purely psychological factors.

In the next chapter, we will be looking at other factors that may influence outcome after injury to the head and ways to respond to and manage ongoing symptoms.

3

Understanding the impact and role of other factors

A question that frequently comes up in clinical and research settings is how can the same type of injury happen to two people but have very different effects and outcomes? My answer to this is that we are all unique in terms of genetic make-up, life experiences, health status, belief systems and coping styles. All these factors interplay on many different levels and have a unique impact on how our brain and mind respond and interact with the world, which creates a rich diversity in terms of outcome.

In this chapter we will explore and seek to understand the impact and role of a range of other factors on someone's function and health status in the short term and long term after an injury to the head:

- Pre-existing concussions/injury
- Male vs female
- Other health conditions
- Trauma
- Socio-economic factors
- Beliefs/rules for living
- Ways of interaction with self, others and the world.

Pre-existing head injuries/concussions

A number of my clients (but not all) report a history of previous head trauma due to a variety of causes, be that sport, road traffic accidents, falls or violence. These are injuries that may have happened in their adult life or during childhood. However, while they may not have persistent symptoms following those head injuries, their brain and nervous system have been put under strain and so are vulnerable to further stress and injury. In some cases, the individual may have had an injury where there was no mention of involvement of head or neck; it could be that their back or lower limbs were injured. However, depending on the mechanism of injury, their head may have been subjected to acceleration and deceleration forces, but concussion symptoms did not appear at that time.

Many semi- and professional sports people are subjected to what is known as multiple 'subconcussive' injuries due to the very nature of their sport. We are learning more about the long-term impact of multiple (albeit what appear to be innocuous) injuries to the head and brain, which has meant that governing sports bodies are much more aware of the risk of head trauma and are working towards making contact sport as safe as possible. While helmets in sport protect against physical damage to the skull, the brain within the skull can still be affected for reasons described in Chapter 1. One of the main messages to come out of research into head injuries in sport is to limit the potential of second impact injuries, which can be fatal. As such, if someone has an injury to the head during a sporting event such as rugby or football, the safest thing to do for that player is to immediately send them off the pitch and give them at least two weeks of no contact sport, reducing the chance of second impact syndrome. While on the surface someone might look fine after a knock to the head or upper body, and pass simple pitch-side tests, their brain and sensory system may not be as alert and quick as they need to be to dodge a tackle and they are more likely to be involved in further injury.

Other health conditions

If someone is in poor or suboptimal physical health, it is likely that they may suffer greater impact from a head injury, or any injury for that matter. For example, autoimmune disorders (such as rheumatoid arthritis or coeliac disease) can mean that a person would take longer to recover compared to someone without a pre-existing health condition.

There has been some research looking at the possible association between post-concussion symptoms and Ehlers-Danlos syndrome (EDS). EDS is the name for a group of rare inherited conditions (of which there are 13) that affect people in different ways. The most common type is Hypermobile EDS but other types include classical EDS, vascular EDS and kyphoscoliotic EDS. Common symptoms include hypermobility and issues with connective tissue. Connective tissues provide support within skin, tendons, ligaments, blood vessels, internal organs and bones. Having this condition affects a few different aspects of how someone's body functions and many people with this condition experience pain in their joints. There are several different types of EDS that may share some symptoms, including:

- an increased range of joint movement (joint hypermobility)
- stretchy skin
- fragile skin that breaks or bruises easily
- wounds being slower to heal
- fatiguing more easily
- problem with bladder control.

The issue of hypermobility, weaker connective tissue, reduced neck strength and cervical instability has been linked to a greater vulnerability to the impact of a concussion, as well as reduced or slowed recovery following one. This is hypothesized to be due to the head of someone with EDS being less protected by cervical structure. Some researchers have suggested that people presenting with persistent symptoms after a head injury should undergo a thorough review of their symptom so that an underlying diagnosis of Ehlers-Danlos syndrome is not overlooked.

Unfortunately, there is no specific treatment for EDS, the focus is more on the management of symptoms. People with

EDS may benefit from seeking input from a physiotherapist to learn exercises to strengthen joints and avoid injuries, an occupational therapist to advise on management of daily activities as well as fatigue, and psychological support if the person is struggling to cope with the symptoms. However, there is some indication that oxygen therapy may provide some benefit as it has been found to provide the following:

- faster healing
- energy boosts
- reduced pain
- decreased swelling and inflammation
- combatting of infection.

As with living with any chronic condition, treatment is about creating balance between looking after yourself and engaging in activities that do not cause harm, but not being so restrictive that you cannot lead a healthy, well-rounded life.

More information regarding EDS can be found below:

- Ehlers-Danlos Support UK – you can also call their free helpline on 0800 907 8518, find local support groups or visit their online forum.
- Hypermobility Syndromes Association (HMSA) – you can also call their helpline on 0333 011 6388, find local groups or visit their online forum.

Male vs female

'Sex' refers to a set of biological attributes in humans and animals that are dependent on chromosomes, hormone levels and reproductive anatomy. 'Gender' meanwhile refers to behavioural expressions, socially constructed roles, expressions and identities which intersect with sex and other determinants of health. As such, exploring the complex and interconnected role of sex and gender in an injury or illness is a challenge.

For the purpose of this section, I will look at the broad difference between males and females in terms of risk factors, impact and outcome from mTBI, as a way of exploring *why* there may be differences.

It appears from a number of studies that females sustain concussions more frequently than males and subsequently have more severe neurological symptoms that take longer to resolve. There may be a number of reasons for these differences which include anatomical differences in the neck and head/neck stability that make females more vulnerable to injury, as well as different biomechanical thresholds (i.e. the level of force needed to cause an injury).

A newer line of exploration has been into hormonal factors, which can be affected by head and neck injury. Given that structures in the centre of the brain responsible for regulating the body's hormonal release (e.g. hypothalamus and/pituitary gland) are also frequently affected during an acceleration/deceleration injury, there is an increasing recognition of the role of changes in hormonal levels in symptom manifestation and presentation. The range and overlap between the effects of injury to the hypothalamus and pituitary gland and effects of brain injury are huge and varied (e.g. mood swings, change in sex drive, fatigue, headaches, altered body temperature, weight gain, change in menstrual cycle), so it can be difficult to tease out what is due to brain injury and what is due to hormonal changes, which can result in hypopituitarism. While it is not standard practice to refer for specialist hormonal tests following a head injury, clinicians (e.g. GPs and neurologists) are becoming increasingly aware of the value of further endocrine investigations in order to explore potential hormonal treatment options to assist in someone's recovery. Some studies have looked at how the phase of the menstrual cycle a woman is in when she has a concussion can impact recovery outcomes, due to changes in hormonal levels, specifically in the reduction of progesterone concentration.

Progesterone effects on the reproductive and endocrine systems are well known but more recent studies have found it has neuro-protective effects on the central nervous system, of which the brain is part. That is, it can improve functional recovery by protecting or rebuilding the blood–brain barrier, decreasing development of cerebral edema, down-regulating the inflammatory cascade and limiting loss of neural tissue. Female hormones such as oestrogen may have a role in pain response and experience in females compared to males.

Another new and important research finding has suggested that the differences in the thickness of white matter structure in men and women may explain why more women may suffer persisting symptoms and outcome after an injury to the head compared to men.

There are of course other factors that make females more vulnerable to having a head injury and subsequent mTBI. Sadly, violence against women is a big part of this. Women are more likely to be subjected to assault and injury (physical, psychological and emotional) by intimate partners as well as being victims of abuse in childhood. We'll look at the impact of childhood trauma on brain development and vulnerability below.

Pink Concussions <https://www.pinkconcussions.com/> is a US-based non-profit organization that focuses on pre-injury education and post-injury medical care for women and girls with brain injury, including concussion incurred from sport, violence, accidents or military service. The website has a host of content and resources. The founder, Katherine Snedaker, and her team are very passionate about changing the current identification, management and support of women and girls with brain injuries.

Trauma and pre-existing psychological issues

There has been an amazing level of growth in our understanding of trauma, which is reflected not only in how it is diagnosed and classified but also in terms of how it is treated.

We now know that trauma does not need to be to the level where it reaches a diagnosis of Post-Traumatic Stress Disorder (PTSD) but can be present if the individual has experienced disrupted attachment relationships with caregivers in childhood, parental neglect, as well as more obvious and well-known traumatic experiences such as physical and sexual abuse. Complex or development PTSD (c-PTSD) is now being recognized as a cumulation of traumatic experiences that start in childhood. Lead clinicians are even calling for the diagnosis 'borderline personality disorder' (BPD), which is a psychiatric diagnosis, to be better understood as complex PTSD. This shift in perspective and diagnosis serves to understand that the person who has previously been labelled with BPD is highly likely to have suffered extreme trauma. How they function in day-to-day life and interact with others is a manifestation of coping strategies (albeit maladaptive) that their brain and mind have developed to deal with the toxic levels of stress they have in their nervous system as a result of the distressing things that happened to them, usually in childhood.

Some eminent trauma experts such as Gabor Maté, Bessel van der Kolk and Peter Levine have spent their long careers looking at what trauma is and how it affects individuals, families and society. On an individual level, trauma can affect the structure of the brain. Research has shown that the brain develops differently in a child who experiences trauma compared to those that do not. It has been found that there are variations in volume and surface area of the insula, which is a region of the brain buried deep in the cerebral cortex that is crucial for self-awareness and reaction to sensory information. Subcortical white matter has also been found to be less robust and so potentially more sensitive to physical injury.

Adults who have not received treatment to help them with traumatic experiences they have had as children are more likely to suffer from mental health issues such as anxiety and depression. When adults have experienced trauma and have been diagnosed with PTSD, neuroimaging studies have found certain areas of the brain to be affected, such as the amygdala, the hippocampus and the ventromedial prefrontal cortex (vmPFC). The amygdala is sometimes termed the 'fear centre of the brain' as it is thought of as the core of the neural system for processing fearful and threatening stimuli, including detection of threat and activation of appropriate fear-related behaviours in response to danger. It is also part of the system that integrates emotion into memories.

The hippocampus is a part of another system in the brain involved in memory processing and differentiating between past and present experiences. When someone is exposed to a traumatic event, the hippocampus can be flooded with cortisol (stress hormone), which then affects the functioning and potentially even the volume of the hippocampus. As a result, people may have trouble working out, on a cognitive level, the difference between past threats and their current situation, which can lead to behavioural avoidance of everyday situations and activities that they may perceive as threatening (e.g. social interaction, leisure activities, being in public spaces). This is because the memory of past trauma is ever present and so influences motivation to step into these scenarios. Behavioural avoidance reinforces the notion that activities are challenging/dangerous as it is never disproved, and people become more and more hyper-vigilant to potential threat as a biological safety mechanism. Also due to the amygdala being continually activated, a bigger neural network is created, which increases the volume of the amygdala. This has a negative impact on mood and the ability to control emotions as when the amygdala is activated, it shuts down the rational thinking part of the brain that is the prefrontal cortex (PFC). As a result, the PFC loses volume and controlling reactions and behaviour becomes more difficult. A vicious cycle ensues for the individual where they feel on high alert to threat and engage in avoidance of situations, which means their nervous system becomes less and less able to deal with stress. How does this relate to mTBI and PCS? We'll look at this shortly.

The late Dr Robert Scaer was a wonderful neurologist who spent a lot of his clinical life exploring people who had poor outcomes after what were traditionally known as whiplash injuries. In his first book, *The Body Bears the Burden*, he explores how individuals who have experienced ruptured childhood attachments then go on to have disrupted boundaries, which then results in a heightened physical and psychological response to further experiences of rupture to their boundaries such as an abrupt physical trauma like being in a car crash.

For many years the link between previous mental health issues and worse outcomes after a TBI/head injury has been strongly postulated. Many identify pre-injury psychological issues as a vulnerability factor to experiencing psychological issues and delayed recovery after an injury to the head. In my view, this notion that 'if you were depressed and/or anxious before an injury then you are more likely to be depressed/anxious after it' is a simplistic explanation. Why would someone develop depression and/or anxiety in the first place? Are depression and anxiety a result of childhood trauma that was never dealt with, did the childhood trauma impact on how the brain developed? This takes us back to the argument that psychological trauma causes physical changes in the brain, which means the brain of someone who has suffered trauma is potentially less robust to deal with further neuro-trauma, that is a concussion and mTBI. In my view, vulnerability can be understood as occurring through a combination of pathophysiological and psychological pre-injury status.

The role of epigenetics is also being identified as playing an important role in our health. In other words, while our genes play a significant part in our health status, so does what we do (e.g. how we eat, exercise and think), as well as our environment and experiences. Epigenetics studies how our behaviours and environment can cause changes that affect the way our genes work and these changes are passed down to children. Unlike genetic changes, epigenetic changes are reversible and do not change our DNA sequence, but they can change how our body reads a DNA sequence. It has been found that parents' stressful experiences can influence their children's vulnerability to many pathological conditions, including medical conditions and psychiatric illness, and their effects may even endure for several generations. An example of this was found with the children of Holocaust survivors. While these individuals had not been in concentration camps and were born after the war, researchers found that they were experiencing trauma symptoms despite not being directly exposed to it. Of course, this feeds into the nature/nurture debate and you could argue that such transmission of trauma was caused by environmental factors, that is, the parents not being able to function as secure attachment bases to their children due to their traumatic experiences. However, it is also possible that these children were 'marked' epigenetically with a chemical coating on their chromosomes, a biological memory from the experience of their parents which made them less able to deal with and more vulnerable to stress. Integrating both hereditary and environmental factors as well as epigenetics adds a new dimension to the explanation of transgenerational transmission of trauma.

Socio-economic factors

Socio-economic status (along with race and ethnicity) affects people's access to education, adequate nutrition, well-being resources, as well as the ability to access services that they may need. Lower socio-economic status has been linked not only to a higher likelihood of experiencing a head injury and subsequent brain injury, but also to a poorer outcome.

Those living in deprivation are more likely to be subjected to traumatic experiences in childhood. The wonderful work of Dr Nadine Burke Harris looks at the connection of childhood adversity and long-term health status. The principle is that adversity has direct and indirect effects on someone's physical health. In her book *The Deepest Well: Healing the Long-term Effects of Childhood Adversity*, she fully explores the biology underlying the connection between adverse childhood experiences (ACEs) and poor health status, both physical and psychological.

Beliefs and rules for living

You may be someone who has never really had an injury, or someone who feels that to overcome an injury, you have to push on through. I have seen this in many of my clients who feel that they can get over a brain injury by exercising it like an injured muscle. However, a brain injury is far more complex than a leg or shoulder injury. From a clinical point of view, this approach can serve as a hindrance rather than a help with this type of injury, as it disallows recognition of ongoing symptoms in a way that facilitates physical and psychological accommodation to be made.

In clinic, we see this in people who are very goal focused and used to achieving by pushing their body and mind to the limit. While this is traditionally seen in professional sports people, this way of living, rooted in competition, seems to be becoming the norm. We are all living hectic, busy lives that have no margin for error, so having an injury that slows us down is seen as a massive disadvantage and potentially a weakness, not only on an individual but also on a societal level. Such a lifestyle has a direct effect on our autonomic nervous system, in that we are more in sympathetic activation than parasympathetic activation. This means our nervous system is 'stretched' and more activated to respond in sympathetic mode. If the nervous system was more balanced, and the time spent being in parasympathetic or dorsal ventral mode was increased, there would be more capacity to recover. I will be linking this to self-management techniques in later sections.

4

Differential diagnosis

In healthcare, differential diagnosis uses your history along with presenting issues and symptoms to arrive at the correct diagnosis. The aim is to use a mode of deduction to distinguish a particular illness, disease or condition from others that present with similar clinical features. In medical and psychiatric practice, this approach is used to systematically identify the presence of a disease or diagnosis where multiple alternatives are possible. It is a process of testing a hypothesis relating to a clinical presentation, medical knowledge and case history. In the fields of psychiatry and psychology, there is often a big overlap between diagnoses as so many symptoms can present themselves in multiple conditions. This sometimes means that patients can be given a range of different diagnoses by different doctors depending on where the doctor focuses their clinical attention the most, in light of the specific field they work in, their clinical experience, research interests and even country of training. While differential diagnosis is a high-level clinical skill, unfortunately it can be affected by a range of conscious and unconscious human biases.

In my years of working with a range of clients after a head injury, I have come across various different diagnoses apart from mTBI and post-concussion syndrome, which I will briefly outline below.

Post-traumatic stress disorder (PTSD)

In terms of symptomatology there is a big overlap between PTSD and mTBI. There is a range of opinion as to whether they can co-exist or whether one diagnosis trumps the other. Often people diagnosed with a concussion and/or mTBI have minimal loss of consciousness, which means they often have recollection immediately prior to the event, less recall of the actual point of impact, but then recall of the aftermath. Usually, all these points surrounding the event were likely to have been quite traumatic and potentially life threatening (i.e. road traffic accident, a fall or assault). I have heard multiple descriptions from clients describing the high levels of fear and/or helplessness they experienced just before an accident or injury. For example, some have told me that they saw another car approaching and could do nothing but 'brace' themselves, or that they 'froze' and felt 'time slow down'. Some people even describe the phenomenon of their life flashing before their eyes, due to thinking that they are going to die. Others who may have lost consciousness briefly and then 'came round' after the injury describe experiencing confusion and shock initially, especially if they found themselves trapped in a car. This may be an unfounded generalization but anecdotally, I have found that females I see tell me that after an accident or injury, they tend to not want to make a fuss, they often just want to carry on or get home, feeling embarrassed by the fact they have been involved in an accident or been hurt. Males, meanwhile, tend to report more anger. Both men and women describe symptoms of shock, which is protective in the very short term as adrenaline is released into the body. This then serves as anaesthesia so that the pain of soft tissue injuries may not be experienced immediately, but being in a state of shock can be very dangerous for an individual if prolonged, as the body goes into shutdown.

In terms of ongoing symptoms after a traumatic injury, people can experience intrusions in the form of flashbacks and nightmares, hyperarousal (demonstrated by feeling 'on edge'), being physically agitated, having reduced concentration and sleep disturbance, as well as psychological and behavioural avoidance. They might try to block out thoughts of the event or situations that remind them of the event/injury and avoid going near where the injury occurred or situations that are familiar. People talk to me about taking different routes so that they do not have to walk near the place where the accident occurred, or they avoid driving if the accident occurred in a vehicle. However, people with more severe brain injuries where the period of being unconscious was longer and who have no memory of the event, before it or some time after it, can also have a similar range of symptoms associated with PTSD. With regards to the overlap of symptoms between brain injury and PTSD, when an individual has suffered trauma physically, psychosocially and neurologically, as commonly experienced in road traffic accidents, falls, assaults and combat, disentangling the symptoms and trying to dichotomize them as being caused by either PTSD or brain injury is a differential diagnosis challenge because so many of the symptoms are shared.

In the many cases I have worked with where a diagnosis of PTSD is given, some individuals are referred for and take part in evidence-based, trauma-focused psychological therapy. While this psychological intervention does help with processing the traumatic thoughts and feelings, and people experience a reduction in or amelioration of distressing dreams and flash-backs, they continue to have cognitive symptoms. These might include poor concentration, reduced memory and difficulty with decision making, as well as somatic symptoms of ongoing sleep disturbance and fatigue. This supports the position that both conditions can exist together and treating PTSD is very helpful for mTBI and PCS and should constitute a part of the holistic treatment package as it helps to 'clear' some of the emotional distress and feelings of overwhelm. The person can start to engage in more behavioural strategies in an effort to return to day-to-day activities, as they are not as inhibited by the symptoms associated with trauma.

Mood and anxiety disorders

In terms of the post-injury mood/emotional/affective symptoms, the emerging research proposes three major pathways/mechanisms at play as detailed below.

- **Immediate psychological injury:** although TBI does not cause PTSD, some people, particularly those who were conscious in the aftermath of the injury and experienced the event and injury as life threatening, are likely to suffer an acute stress response, which puts them at high risk of PTSD. This factor alone has a negative impact on outcome. Sometimes the trauma they experience in the injury activates other possibly unresolved traumatic experiences. For most patients, without the insult to the brain the trauma response would be much less, if present at all. For experiences of trauma without brain injury, psychological treatment tends to be much more effective, and clients are not left with the residual TBI symptoms of fatigue, light and noise sensitivity and cognitive deficits.

- **Brain-based insult secondary to white matter injury:** there is increasing recognition that a significant proportion of symptoms may be directly attributable to white matter injury in TBI (and other neurological conditions), especially when mood disturbance is seen immediately after the injury. The link between inflammation and neuropsychiatric diagnosis is increasingly recognized and may be closely intertwined and possibly working together in a bidirectional loop where depression causes inflammation, but, equally, inflammation promotes depression and other neuropsychiatric disorders. An important factor in identifying what came first is the timeline of injury and symptoms evolution. Often people describe their mood to be low immediately after the injury, which would point to the inflammation causing the mood disturbance rather than the other way around. Of course, over time, as detailed below, this becomes a vicious cycle.

- **Reactive, secondary psychological injury:** many individuals experience neuropsychiatric symptoms such as anxiety and depression in response to the struggle and difficulty they have in daily life as a result of the cognitive and functional compromise that ensues following the injury. This can bring up feelings of shame, guilt, frustration and worry as they find they are unable to function as they did prior to the injury. There are also psychological reactions to loss of role, relationships and employment in many cases. In clinic, I see clients that have experienced a series of losses following an mTBI which can include physical stamina, mental agility, social acumen, status within the family, leadership roles in work and standing in social circles.

Also, to clarify, in those individuals whose depression is diagnosed without a recent injury to the head and/or brain, it is the depression that can, in some cases, but not all, cause the cognitive problems of poor concentration, attention, memory and slowed processing speed. The symptoms of fatigue, disrupted sleep pattern, poor concentration and avoidance of social interaction can appear to be, and often are, misdiagnosed as depression but are symptoms in their own right and very common after brain injury.

All the three pathways we've seen above may well be working together to cause the persistent presence of post-injury psychological difficulties. These, in combination with the post-injury specific cognitive weaknesses, will have a negative impact on how someone interacts with the world.

When I talk about pre-injury mental health issues with my clients in clinic, a proportion of people (as would be the case with the general population) have experienced mental health issues, be that anxiety and/or low mood. Some may have had treatment for mental health disorders and found it beneficial. However, while many may have been diagnosed as experiencing anxiety and depression post-injury (usually by their GP, due to the description of their symptoms), people often reflect that what they experience post-injury feels different in comparison. Also, that pre-injury, while they may have been suffering from mental health issues, they were able to function within their job and manage the demands of everyday life. This points to the fact that what they are experiencing post-injury is more than a purely mental health issue.

Anna told me that pre-injury, she had experienced a short period of anxiety when she was in her early 20s that had no impact on her ability to work. Post-injury the anxiety she felt was very different, both in severity and in its persistence and impact on her life. She gave the example of a time, around three months after her concussion, when in an attempt to get back to normal life, she had decided to drive her children to a local theatre to see a children's show. However, just as she was at a large roundabout, she experienced what could be classified as a panic attack. Anna describes her experience below.

Box 3. Anna's experience of panic

The first panic attack was like a huge uncontrollable wave that came out of nowhere. I was overcome with fear and terror. I wanted to do the correct thing, i.e. drive my car, yet, at the same time, I felt paralyzed. Also, I felt this experience not just as an emotional one but as a physical one. It felt as if a huge surge of electricity was going through my body in the place where my physical soft tissue injuries were, i.e. from my head down the right hand side of my body, down my neck, shoulder, arm and back, and right leg. On reflection, it was as if my system was overwhelmed by all the different stimuli and the act of having to concentrate hard and do multiple things at once. Fortunately, there was a police station close, so I drove there and turned up on the doorstep in tears. I felt very embarrassed as we had to be driven home by two policemen.

I had further panic attacks over the next few days. One was when my husband was driving us down a country road and some motor-bikes overtook us. I experienced something similar to the previous panic attack. My heart was pounding like crazy and the noise of the bikes roared through my head and terrified me. It was as if I was having a nightmare. I think it was the next day that I went to see my GP about these experiences. Both while in the waiting room and while sitting next to him as he took my blood pressure, I experienced these bizarre feelings of intense anxiety and overwhelm again, both emotionally and physically. I ended up crying in front of the doctor. It was so weird and I felt that I had no control over my emotions, the physical sensations or what was happening to me. I'd never experienced anything like it before. A couple of times previously in my life, many years prior to my accident, I'd felt anxious, but it was not on the same scale, nor did it have that overwhelming emotional and physical intensity. Previously it had been a case of a specific situation triggering me to feel anxious, followed by a narrative running through my head of 'this is uncomfortable, I don't like it, I need to avoid this'. It eventually subsided and disappeared. It wasn't sharp, very intense, and like an overwhelming shock.

On a subsequent visit to my GP a few months later regarding panic attacks as well as other ongoing symptoms (including headaches, dizziness, being off balance, forgetfulness, slower thinking) I showed him a pamphlet about post-concussion syndrome from the brain injury charity Headway. He gave me a booklet about anxiety and suggested I attend anxiety management classes (which I was unable to do due to distance, inability to drive and childcare commitments). He prescribed me the antidepressant Fluoxetine, which calmed the anxiety for a few months but made me feel drowsy and numb, so I asked for advice on weaning myself slowly off it. I was also prescribed Amitriptyline to help me sleep. I later found out that the GP had written in my notes that he thought I had 'adjustment disorder'. However, he did not inform me of this diagnosis at the time of the consultation.

Psychology professionals who work in mental health settings have very little knowledge and training on neuro conditions and disorders like mTBI and as a result, of course, they find it hard to attribute the symptoms that individuals present to them to anything other than a mental health disorder. People may get a whole host of diagnoses including mood disorder, agoraphobia, social anxiety and panic disorder due to the overlap in symptomatology between mental health disorders and mTBI and PCS. However, the physical and somatic symptoms that people experience after a head injury need to be factored into the differential diagnosis, as people with a purely psychological diagnosis tend to not experience balance problems and sensory issues such as light and noise sensitivity, and changes to smell and taste.

Even for those individuals who have received a diagnosis of mTBI, there is still a propensity among some clinicians to avoid associating ongoing symptoms with mTBI due to the outdated view that this severity of injury does not produce any significant or persistent neuropsychological issues past the three-month point. There has been a tendency to attribute any cognitive deficits to disturbances in emotional functioning and psychological factors (stress, depression and anxiety). However, a number of very recent pieces of scientific research, including the seminal TRACK-TBI study published in 2018, have started to unpick and explore persisting neurocognitive and neurobehavioural issues following a TBI classified as 'mild'. The study has a large sample (over 1000), control group (orthopaedic comparison) and long-term follow-up (12 months). The researchers found that 53 per cent of the mTBI group reported persistent symptoms 12 months post-injury compared to 38 per cent of the orthopaedic trauma group. It is critical to point out that the TRACK-TBI study included both those individuals with changes identified on brain scans and those with scans reported as normal or negative. In fact, over 800 patients had negative scans but reported very similar TBI symptoms and levels of disability to the scan-positive patients. These findings challenge the long-held legal belief that brain injury needs to be evident on a scan in order to be proved, and the long-held medical belief that symptoms of mTBI should resolve in three months and those that do not are psychological rather than organic.

In summary, many people are diagnosed with anxiety and depression as these symptoms are more readily known to GPs and have an evidence base for treatment. However, for people with an mTBI and PCS, while they do present with mood symptoms, the other more physical symptoms are more likely to be ignored as they do not fit nicely into the 'mental health disorder' box. In Anna's case, her GP had never heard of a concussion resulting in visual problems, so she was advised to see an optician (who is focused on vision) rather than a specialist in eye care (an ophthalmologist).

Adjustment disorder

When I first started to get referrals to see people with ongoing symptoms following a head injury, they often came with a diagnosis of adjustment disorder, which can be found in both the DSM-5 and ICD-10. The DSM-5 descriptor is as follows:

A. The development of emotional or behavioural symptoms in response to an identifiable stressor(s) occurring within three months of the onset of the stressor(s)

B. The symptoms or behaviours are clinically significant as evidenced by one or both of the following:

i) Marked distress that is out of proportion to the severity or intensity of the stressor, taking into account the external context and the cultural factors that might influence symptom severity and presentation.

ii) Significant impairment in social, occupational, or other important areas of functioning.

C. The stress-related disturbance does not meet the criteria for another mental disorder and is not merely an exacerbation of a pre-existing mental disorder.

D. The symptoms do not represent normal bereavement.

E. Once the stressor (or its consequence) has terminated, the symptoms do not persist for more than an additional six months.

Whereas the ICD-10 describes the following:

States of subjective distress and emotional disturbance, usually interfering with social functioning and performance, arising in the period of adaptation to a significant life change or a stressful life event. The stressor may have affected the integrity of an individual's social network (bereavement, separation experiences) or the wider system of social supports and values (migration, refugee status), or represented a major developmental transition or crisis (going to school, becoming a parent, failure to attain a cherished personal goal, retirement). Individual predisposition or vulnerability plays an important role in the risk of occurrence and the shaping of the manifestations of adjustment disorders, but it is nevertheless assumed that the condition would not have arisen without the stressor. The manifestations vary and include depressed mood, anxiety or worry (or mixture of these), a feeling of inability to cope, plan ahead, or continue in the present situation, as well as some degree of disability in the performance of daily routine. Conduct disorders may be an associated feature, particularly in adolescents. The predominant feature may be a brief or prolonged depressive reaction, or a disturbance of other emotions and conduct.

While the event that causes the injury is often very stressful and people present with symptoms of anxiety, depression as well as marked distress and impairment in areas of functioning, the level of distress is rarely out of proportion considering the potential life-threatening nature of the event that caused the injury. People may have been thrown off motorbikes or hit by cars mounting the pavement or had something fall on their face from a height. People's inability to function normally is caused by multiple factors, not just by distress, and is made much worse by the cognitive issues happening from changes in the brain. Just like the primary mental health disorders, this diagnosis takes no account of the physical symptoms.

Migraines and post traumatic headaches

Headache is the most common symptom that people report after an injury to the head both in the acute (up to three months) and chronic phases (over three months). The two most common classifications of primary headache are migraine and tension-type headaches (TTH).

Migraine is a neurovascular condition defined by attacks of moderate to severe throbbing headache. It is often accompanied by sensitivities, mostly to light and sound (photophobia and phonophobia) but can also include sensitivity to odour and movement. Some people experience a range of symptoms with migraine such as gastrointestinal symptoms as well as changes in emotional, cognitive and autonomic and vestibular status. To be diagnosed with a chronic migraine, the migraine needs to occur more than 14 days per month, for three months. Sometimes people may have experienced the odd migraine prior to the injury, which would be termed 'episodic', but head trauma has been identified as a possible trigger for transformation from episodic to chronic migraine.

Tension-type headaches are the most prevalent headache disorder in the general population. These are less severe and debilitating than a migraine and have no associated symptoms or features. Although tension-type headaches are common, the pathophysiology and likely mechanism remain unclear. Current knowledge of the nociceptive (pain receptor) system suggests that the pain of tension-type headaches has a muscular origin. This is because the pain typically radiates in a band-like fashion bilaterally from the forehead to the occiput. Pain also often radiates to the neck muscles and is described as tightness, pressure, or dull ache. Unlike migraine, there seems to be only a minor role of hereditary and genetic factors in episodic TTH.

Post traumatic headaches are classified as a secondary type of headache as the causation is directly linked to an organic disease or recognized as a symptom of a recognized disease process. It is hypothesized that a TBI activates an underlying TTH or migraine headache predisposition or it accentuates headaches patterns that were pre-existent to the trauma.

While the literature suggests that many peoples' post traumatic headaches improve over time, there are those that are left with debilitating headaches that are strongly associated with light sensitivity that impact on all aspects of their life and can be challenging for clinicians to treat. Thankfully, more people who are suffering with headaches after a mTBI and are being sent to see neurologists who specialize in the identification and treatment of Post Traumatic Headaches. This means individuals have a better chance of specialist treatment which may not have occurred if their headaches were diagnosed solely as migraine or tension-type and treated only via their primary care physician.

Chronic pain

Often, people with a mTBI experience injuries to other parts of their body, most frequently their neck, shoulders and back. Injuries can be soft tissue and/or nerve related and subsequently cause pain. The pain often goes beyond the acute period and becomes chronic. Chronic pain is pain that lasts more than three months following an injury and as such, can interfere with all aspects of daily life.

Studies have shown that <u>chronic pain</u> may not only be caused by physical injury, but also by <u>stress</u> and emotional factors, and that the relationship is bi-directional. In particular, people who have experienced trauma and suffer from symptoms associated with <u>PTSD</u>, are often at a higher risk of developing chronic pain. Chronic pain is defined as "prolonged physical pain that lasts for longer than the natural healing process should allow". Chronic pain can debilitate one's ability to move with ease and may hinder normal day-to-day functioning, which then results in feelings of anger, hopelessness, <u>depression</u> and anxiety as well as having a detrimental impact on self-esteem. The use of pain medications, while initially may serve as relief, become less efficient as time progresses.

During a traumatic event, the nervous system goes into survival mode and the sympathetic nervous system is activated. If the nervous system stays in survival mode (sympathetic activation) and is not able to revert to a state of balance by activation of the parasympathetic branch of autonomic nervous system, then the body and brain remains in a high tense and alert mode. This mode is helpful in the short term but dysfunctional in the long term, as it causes fatigue and an excess of stress <u>hormones</u> such as cortisol to be released into the bloodstream. Excess cortisol causes an increase in blood pressure and blood sugar, which in turn, can reduce the strength of the immune system and cause stress on other bodily systems, such as the respiratory and cardiovascular systems. Also, high levels of cortisol in the brain can have a detrimental impact on cognitive functioning, especially memory. As such, interventions to assist the individual to regain balance in their nervous system can have a wide ranging and positive impact on the experience of pain. These interventions usually involve mind-body based approaches to foster a sense of safety in one's body, rather than relying on talking therapies alone.

Box 4. Anna details her experience of pain and approaches to treatment

I was referred to see a chronic pain specialist at my local hospital who was happy that the steps I was taking with physiotherapy and diet were adequate for managing my pain symptoms.

A year after my injury, I saw a new GP for a referral to a private consultant for an upright MRI scan on my back as I was still in pain every day and by that point I was walking with a stick. I thought there must be something very wrong but the scan came back with no remarkable findings. I was grateful that my new doctor had a holistic outlook to healing. Although I think I seemed a bit of a mystery to him, he supported me well and I'm grateful for his care at that time. He referred me to an NHS physiotherapist and later an osteopath who encouraged me to take a lifestyle-based approach to my recovery.

Chronic Fatigue Syndrome (CFS)

CFS or as it was previously known, Myalgic encephalomyelitis (ME) is seen as a complicated disorder that results in the experience of severe and persistent levels of fatigue. It has to have been present for at least six months to reach a diagnosis threshold. It affects the nervous and immune systems and can be sometimes diagnosed as post viral fatigue syndrome (PVFS).

The fatigue associated with CFS is very different to feeling tired. People find they are not able to recover after small levels of physical or mental exertion and sleep or rest does not have an impact on symptoms, which can vary from person to person but can include:

- fatigue
- problems with memory or concentration
- headaches
- sore throat
- enlarged lymph nodes in your neck or armpits

- unexplained muscle or joint pain
- dizziness that worsens with moving from lying down or sitting to standing
- unrefreshing sleep
- extreme exhaustion after physical or mental exercise.

Given that fatigue is also a very common and debilitating symptom associated with all severities of TBI as well as PCS, it is understandable that people may be diagnosed with CFS given the overlap in symptoms. While CFS is a complicated disorder, it can't yet be fully explained by an underlying medical condition, whereas the fatigue after a mTBI and in PCS can be attributed to pathophysiological changes in the brain caused by neuro-trauma. Fatigue after a mTBI is the result of the extra effort the injured brain has to use in processing, assimilating and responding to sensory information and input. When the injured brain becomes overloaded with sensory information, it can result in an acute stress response (activation of sympathetic branch of the nervous system) which can show itself as agitation or aggression (i.e. fight) or needing to get away or avoid (i.e. flight) and in some extreme cases, shutting down (i.e. freeze) as the sense of overload is experienced as threat. This uses up more energy and people feel depleted more quickly and overstimulated in situations that previously did not have such an impact on them. Over time, these experiences of not being adept in dealing with stimulation of everyday life (e.g. public transport, supermarkets, restaurants, bars, work places) results in necessary curbing of activities that put a drain on resources in order to reduce potential behavioural outbursts or panic attacks. On a simplistic level, fatigue reduces someone's ability to function as they did prior to the injury, which then contributes and exacerbates psychological symptoms such anxiety, frustration and low mood.

While some people may find some solace in receiving a diagnosis of CFS, especially if until that point they have been told that there is nothing wrong with them or that their symptoms and struggles can be explained by anxiety or depression, there is still a lack of comprehensive understanding as to why the is they are experiencing severe fatigue. In addition, the cause of CFS is not fully understood. There are many theories ranging from viral infections to psychological stress and some believe that chronic fatigue syndrome might be triggered by a combination of factors. Unfortunately, in many cases, fatigue after a mTBI can be experienced for many years. The individual has to make choices about what they can and can't engage with in order to preserve energy levels, but at the same time balancing the curbing of activities with maintaining quality of life and personal relationships. For both CFS and fatigue in PCS, treatment tends to take a behavioural approach in terms of identifying common triggers of increased fatigue and noticing them before fatigue gets to a level where people cannot function, pacing to avoid 'boom and bust' cycles, as well as planning activities to allow for rest and restoration. Psychological response is also important, and we'll look at this in Chapter 8.

Functional Neurological Disorder/Syndrome (FND/FNS)

FND refers to neurological symptoms like tremor, weakness in the limbs, loss of feeling in part of the body or changes in sensory processing and blackouts, all of which can be very debilitating and result in significant day-to-day difficulties. However, unlike conditions such as stroke, Parkinson's disease and multiple sclerosis (that can result in similar symptoms) which are associated with structural pathology and lesions in the central nervous system and so are understood as being 'hardware' issues, the symptoms of FND are thought to be a 'software' issue. This means they are not associated with structural abnormality in the CNS.

While there are no standard tests for functional neurological disorder, positive diagnostic features of FND have been identified by neurologists. FND is usually diagnosed by a neurologist or a neuropsychiatrist by what symptoms are present and comparing their pattern and presentation to other neurological or medical conditions in order to rule them out. An FND diagnosis is not just made by what is absent, such as a lack of structural changes on an MRI or abnormalities on an EEG.

In the DSM-5, FND comes under the criteria for conversion disorder and lists the following:

- One or more symptoms that affect body movement or senses.
- Symptoms can't be explained by a neurological or other medical condition or another mental health disorder.
- Symptoms cause significant distress or problems in social, work or other areas, or they are significant enough that medical evaluation is recommended.

While FND has traditionally been understood as more of a software rather than a hardware issue, there is emerging neuroimaging evidence to suggest some individuals with FND do actually have structural alterations in certain parts of the brain, including the fornix and corpus callosum (Diez et al., 2021), as well as in sensorimotor, prefrontal and limbic structures (Bègue et al., 2019). What is yet to be explored fully is whether these structural alterations are pre-existing the FND or a consequence of the disorder. As we detailed in Chapter 2, the white matter can be affected in diffuse axonal injury, which occurs when the head is subjected to external forces. However, white matter integrity and functioning of subcortical brain areas are also affected by childhood trauma and early life adversity. Many trauma experts (mainly in the USA) directly link FND to the effect that psychological trauma and adversity have on the brain, especially the developing one, but the opinion in the UK is that trauma is a risk factor but not a direct cause of FND.

In terms of how this relates to people with a head injury and concussion, some people who have persistent symptoms have been diagnosed as having FND, specifically functional cognitive disorder, given the issues with memory, concentration, decision making, multi-tasking and processing speed. Some clinicians consider these symptoms 'non-specific' but I see this constellation of cognitive symptoms, which are subtly picked up on neuropsychological testing, associated with subcortical brain dysfunction. Neurological conditions that affect subcortical regions, like Parkinson's and vascular dementia, show a similar cognitive profile. As we saw in Chapter 3, the subcortex (white matter) of someone's brain may have been vulnerable to injury if that person suffered experiences that changed the structure and functioning of their brain pre-injury. As we saw in that chapter, the subcortical part of the brain (i.e. white matter) may be less robust if the individual has suffered early life experiences that changed the structure and subsequent functioning of their brain. When this is the case, the brain, particularly the subcortical regions, may have less capacity to withstand and heal from new physical neuro-trauma.

Other terms that have been used over the years in neurology and psychiatry to try to understand and explain a host of symptoms and presentations that are felt to be more 'software' rather than 'hardware' are listed below. What this demonstrates is that diagnoses are not fixed, but can change over time. Diagnostic terms are not only influenced by scientific research but also by social and political factors.

Functional: Implies the problem culminates from a change in function (in the context of FND – the nervous system) rather than structure.

Hysteria: An old term coined by Freud that describes a complex neurosis where psychological conflicts manifest into physical symptoms.

Dissociative disorders: Indicates dissociation as the main mechanism in symptom manifestation. Dissociation has numerous definitions, but in the context of FND refers to two particular phenomena called derealization and depersonalization.

Psychogenic: Suggests that symptoms are psychologically influenced.

Conversion disorder: Proposition based on the idea of conversion from mental distress to physical symptoms.

Health anxiety/Hypochondriasis: Excessive anxiety about the possibility of a serious disease and stressing over minor symptoms. Typically reassurance is sought from medical professionals but the effects are short lived.

Factitious disorder: When people intentionally fabricate symptoms to obtain medical care.

Malingering: Making up symptoms for material gain (healthcare, benefits, compensation).

As a neuropsychologist, my role involves trying to understand the brain and the mind that the injury occurs to, rather than just the injury. I have worked with individuals with a range of neurological conditions, but mTBI is one of the most challenging, mainly due to the age at which it typically occurs, and thus the degree of impact on work, family and social life. Adding the context of the controversy that surrounds it, due to the invisible nature of the injury, it is even harder for the people with brain injury themselves to understand, let alone loved ones and employers. Over time, as I have seen more and more people from a range of backgrounds with a variety of presentations come to my clinic for assessment and treatment, along with exploration of the research (historical and contemporary), as well as sometimes lively discussion and debates with a wide range of colleagues, I have deepened and broadened my understanding of this condition. We should approach each individual story as a curious scientist who does their best to leave biases and judgements outside the clinic door. This position means that we should be able to have our views and hypotheses tested and retested and be open to the vast amount of opinion in the field.

In the book *The Ghost in My Brain* by Dr Clark Elliott, the author documents his concussion and subsequent recovery. He refers to the many letters he has received since the book's publication in 2018. He writes that one doctor, after reading the book, wrote to him and stated,

> 'I am haunted by a vision of the faces of people I have misdiagnosed over the years. These faces stretch far off into the horizon. Over and over I see a person I remember and think, it was a brain injury and I missed it. Never again. Your book has profoundly changed my practice.'

5

What to do in the immediate post-injury phase

It is important to seek early medical attention if you have experienced an injury to the head/face and/or had your head shaken around, as in a crash or a fall. Many people do go to Accident and Emergency (A&E), but usually not immediately because the injury results in a neurometabolic cascade of changes and damage that evolve over minutes, hours and days, rather than an immediate effect. As a result, many people return to their day-to-day lives without taking adequate time off to rest and recover. It is under these conditions (i.e. return to normal work and life routine) that physical, cognitive and emotional symptoms and difficulties can increase and culminate over time. DAI mostly damages the subcortical part of the brain that includes the limbic system, which is the 'seat of emotions'. Emotional symptoms like anxiety, irritability and low mood are as diagnostically relevant as the physical symptoms (e.g. headache, dizziness and sensory sensitivity) and the cognitive symptoms (e.g. reduced concentration, slowed thinking).

During a visit to A&E with a head injury, depending on the clinical assessment recommendations, neuroimaging will be undertaken, most likely a CT scan. In some cases, you could get an MRI, but this is rare. These investigations are to rule out any urgent issues like a bleed or gross structural damage that would require immediate intervention. However, in nine out of ten cases, the images are reported as normal, and patients get sent home with a leaflet advising them to monitor symptoms and to return if their symptoms get worse. Very few people get access to a specialist in concussion from an A&E referral.

Around 80 per cent of people will recover from a head injury or a concussion. This is probably one of the reasons that statutory service provision is limited. Often private sector services look to the NHS for guidelines and an evidence base. There is a lack of specialism in the field and so a lack of drilling down and understanding the specificity of the symptoms in the acute, subacute and chronic phase after a brain injury classified as mild. Most of our understanding about this injury comes from the world of sport and the military (blast injuries). These services have a better developed understanding and are well resourced for assessment and treatment pathways, as well as research. Unfortunately, this is yet to fully trickle down to service provision for the general public.

Many people do visit their GP or family doctor, but as knowledge about mTBI is limited outside of specialist services, it can be hard for these doctors to know how to understand the symptoms that people present with and make a diagnosis. More often than not, doctors prescribe antidepressants and analgesics as the individual usually reports issues with fatigue, concentration and pain. The doctor may make onward referrals to physiotherapy and mental health services in some cases, which can assist the individual with some of their symptoms, but these services usually work in a silo and don't take a joined-up approach to the management of the injury and subsequent symptoms. As there are limited multidisciplinary pathways for assessment, diagnosis and treatment of mTBI, people often have the experience of bouncing around and being sent from pillar to post. While there are small pockets of specialist statutory services, they are incredibly stretched. If the GP does refer the individual to a neurologist, there are long wait lists and when they do get to see the specialist, symptoms may have become chronic. An individual may also need to be referred to other specialist services for investigations such as ophthalmology for visual issues, audio-vestibular physicians for balance and inner ear issues and endocrinologists to look at possible hormonal changes. Again, there is no standardized pathway, at least in the UK, so treatment is very much dependent on the knowledge of the family doctor of this relatively specialist field.

The recent report from the USA *'Traumatic Brain Injury: A Roadmap for Accelerating Progress'* (2022) is a wonderful example of what a small group of highly specialized clinicians are trying hard to implement when it comes to serving people with a TBI:

> In this study most respondents identified a delayed recovery as symptoms or signs persisting after five days in both adults and children. It has been demonstrated in experimental models that concussion injury triggers a neurometabolic cascade of events resulting in abnormal potassium, calcium, glutamate, glucose, and lactate levels and altered cerebral blood flow which takes seven to ten days to resolve. Additional microglial and inflammatory responses can continue for considerably longer than this initial metabolic cascade. If GPs are expecting resolution of symptoms in a concussed patient within five days, it may be that patients are being allowed to return to activities where they risk sustaining a further concussive force too early and this may have clinical consequences. It has been suggested that phase of recovery should be considered in regard to treatment approaches: Acute (0–4 weeks), Post-Acute (4–12 weeks) and Persistent (> 3 months).

The next section will look at things you can do to help self-manage your symptoms in the immediate phase. Please remember that this section is not meant to replace medical advice but to be used in conjunction with it.

First 24–48 hours

You have had an injury to your head/neck/face/upper body. You may or may not have lost consciousness, but you may notice some changes in how you feel. You may experience nausea or sensitivity to light and/or sound. Given your brain may have been injured, giving it rest from unnecessary stimulation will mean it can focus on healing and recovery in this initial window. While I rarely see people this soon after an injury, given my role as a neuropsychologist, I do retrospectively gather as much information as possible on what people did or did not do immediately after the injury. I ask them how they felt, how they responded and if they noticed any symptoms. I also speak to family, friends or work colleagues that may be able to provide more information on whether the individual with the injury had difficulty remembering those initial few days. Gathering a wealth of information from a range of people has allowed me to decipher and pick up patterns of what may or may not help.

As I see people with the whole range of TBI severity in my clinical practice, I have found that those classified as having more significant brain injuries who are treated in hospital immediately after the injury sometimes do not struggle as much with symptoms down the line. This has led me to wonder if this is due to the enforced physical and cognitive rest that an inpatient setting brings, which allows a certain amount of spontaneous brain healing. As such I suggest the following tips may be of benefit in allowing the brain to heal for those people that are not admitted to hospital:

1 Avoid use of screens for at least the first 24 hours.
2 Avoid engaging in high-level thinking and cognitive tasks.
3 Avoid stimulants such as alcohol and coffee.
4 Drink plenty of water.
5 Eat foods that help reduce inflammation (e.g. fresh fruits such as berries, green leafy vegetables, nuts, salmon, olive oil).
6 Speak to your GP about pain relief.
7 Try to have someone with you.
8 Clear your diary – rest your body and brain.
9 Avoid hectic social situations or intense work tasks.

10   Practise gentle self-massage of face, neck and head.
11   Create, as much as possible, a feeling of safety.
12   Do some breathing exercises (e.g. 10 slow deep breaths every three hours).
13   Practise some mindfulness meditation.
14   Do some gentle stretching.

I appreciate that these tips work well in theory, but if you are a parent of young children, a carer, or are in the middle of a specific work task it can be really hard to stop and rest and engage in self-care practices such as these. This list is meant to provide some examples of what you can do to try to allow natural brain healing to happen rather than putting the brain and body under stress while they are trying to recover.

A really interesting experience of someone who was involved in a road traffic accident as a pedestrian is provided by Dr Peter Levine, who is the founder of Somatic Experiencing (SE) and author of many wonderful books including *In an Unspoken Voice*. In this book he details his experience of being knocked over by a car and how, because of his expertise and training, he knew that what he needed in the immediate aftermath of the injury was to feel safe. A sense of safety was provided by a passer-by who happened to be a paediatrician. He asked that she just be with him and that allowed his nervous system to be co-regulated by her calm presence. He also gives the example of another 'helper' who reinforced a sense of fear in him initially rather than safety and the impact this would have potentially had on him if he did not have his knowledge of trauma and trauma treatment. (You can watch Dr Levine talking about this experience in more detail via this link: <https://www.youtube.com/watch?v=9hP2KJ3UgDI>)

This story really emphasizes the role that physical and psychological trauma can have on keeping the nervous system in a state of hyperarousal or sympathetic activation. As we learned in Chapter 1, when we are in fight or flight or freeze our body is unable to heal, rest and restore. Many people have told me how they felt after experiencing the injury. Like Anna, many just wanted to get home or to a place of safety.

Some individuals unfortunately experience stressful inter-actions with others during and after the injury. For example, some individuals have spoken about being shouted at by others (whose error may have caused the injury) after being involved in a road traffic accident. Others have talked about their experience of being in A&E, if they did go to be checked out. Given the head injury is regarded as 'mild' and often there is no obvious external visible injury, and emergency services are so stretched and pressurized, people can feel that they are wasting doctors' and hospital time. In some rare instances, people have felt that A&E doctors have been dismissive of their symptoms, especially if they have attended a few days after the injury when they started to experience an increase or persistence in their symptoms.

48 hours–2 weeks

Scaling back on normal activity in the first two days may be a way of preventing the metabolic cascade of damage. However, there is no research to say this is the case, it is more a hypothesis. For those people that attend A&E, the advice received there can be quite variable. Some of my clients have been told by A&E doctors that they should be fine and to carry on as normal, some were told to engage in 'cognitive rest' for a few days and some were given a leaflet telling them to keep a look out for further symptoms. Many people I see state that they do not know what 'cognitive rest' means. Also, what constitutes rest for one person may equate to being busy for another. This is why strategies need to be bespoke and targeted to the individual.

I recommend keeping a track of symptoms, as this is what helps the individual with the injury and clinicians understand potential triggers to symptoms which can merge and present as panic attacks. This then allows the individual to make adjustments and modifications to reduce the impact of their symptoms. There is the view among some clinicians that tracking symptoms or being overly focused on symptoms can prolong them or even make them worse. The hypothesis is linked to the issues of hypervigilance to bodily sensations that is referred to a lot in the health psychology literature in relation to health anxiety. However, from my experience, people with health anxiety have the propensity to be on high alert to symptoms prior to having an injury and having an injury can exacerbate this tendency. I have only seen this be the case in a few of my clients. I have more often found that people tend to ignore their symptoms after a head injury or explain them away rather than be hypervigilant. For example, I have worked with many individuals who do not pay attention to or ignore symptoms (as they are told to carry on as normal) until it gets to a point that they are overwhelmed by their symptoms and experience what some call a 'relapse' but what I call a 'symptom takedown'. This can be quite an alarming experience as people feel there was no indication as to why they are feeling the way they do. For the individual and the outside world, it does not make sense that they should suddenly have an increase in symptoms, but if they track back the past week, they may have been pushing themselves too far and too fast in their pursuit of normality. In my experience, it is those clients who, prior to the injury, were perhaps used to pushing their bodies to the limit, worked hard to achieve or potentially were not totally in tune with their body and internal sensations, that experience worse symptoms. Part of the work I do with these clients is teaching them to learn to listen to their body in a way they have never done before. I will detail this further in the next section.

During this phase, I would recommend continuing to limit screen time given that screens are very stimulating to our brain and senses and keep us in an aroused state that is not conducive to brain healing. Simply understanding that overstimulation from the environment, a change in blood sugar levels, and pain or increased emotional stress results in an increase in symptoms can help and empower you to make necessary adjustments to reduce the impact of symptoms. Dr Dan Engle in his book *The Concussion Repair Manual* has lots of brilliant resources and information and a section at the back to track symptoms (cognitive, physical, mood and social). I recommend this book to nearly all my clients.

In terms of day-to-day activities, I suggest that people start to slowly build up to more activity but not to the point where their system (body and brain) gets overwhelmed. As we are all different in terms of what commitments and types of activities we do on a daily basis, it would be unhelpful to give a broad statement of what people should or should not do after an injury. As such, I prefer to work in relative terms and speak to clients about doing a percentage less than they were doing pre-injury, while they are in the subacute phase post-injury. So, for the first two weeks think about reducing activity and commitments by at least 50 per cent and monitor symptoms. Continue with the strategies listed above to help rebalance the autonomic nervous system. At this point, you may want to explore body-based interventions that are trauma sensitive. These can range from a lymphatic massage to craniosacral treatment, to acupuncture (if you do not have a needle phobia). Dr Dan Engle recommends using a floatation tank. Engaging in a daily walk in the fresh air and avoiding putting the body and brain under stress with vigorous exercise is recommended. This is so that one can facilitate the parasympathetic branch of the nervous system to be more active in order to promote healing and recovery.

However, given I rarely see people in this acute phase, this recommendation comes from retrospective information gathering from clients. Ideally people would be supported by specialists during this early phase post-injury to minimize further damage and maximize recovery.

2–6 weeks

Applying the above strategies and engaging in a programme of self-care which includes good nutrition, good sleep practices, gentle exercise and autonomic nervous system regulation (which includes restorative practices such as deep and slow breathing, meditation, as well as creating an environment that feel comfortable and safe) will hopefully provide the optimal conditions for healing and recovery. Unfortunately, there are limited prospective research studies on how the application of these sorts of interventions and practices in the acute phase affects outcomes in the long term. Most people are only sent for investigations when they are still suffering with symptoms at the three-month point and by this stage they may have been diagnosed with anxiety, depression and chronic pain rather than post-concussion syndrome or an mTBI. In my view, at this point there has been a missed opportunity for optimizing early recovery.

Symptom-specific strategies

Strategies for physical symptoms:

- Avoid 'boom and bust'.
- Pay attention and notice what your body is telling you.
- Keep track of fatigue.
- Gentle exercise (below symptom threshold).
- Good nutrition.

Strategies for cognitive symptoms:

- Focus on achieving one thing at a time.
- Give yourself more time to complete a task.
- Learn how to say no.
- Create boundaries so that you do not become overloaded.
- Look into using orange-tinted glasses when using screens.

Strategies for psychological symptoms:

- Reduce stress.
- Meditate.
- Pay attention as to who you spend time with.
- Create a nurturing comfortable space.

Strategies for behavioural symptoms:

- Have a daily routine and structure that promotes a balanced day of activity and rest.
- Avoid 'to do' lists, instead mark out time slots in your day to get things done.
- Use the 15-minute principle – just focus on a task for 15 minutes or break tasks down into 15-minute chunks and intersect with regular breaks.

Long-term outcome

Studies have found that a proportion of individuals who experience mTBI have cognitive symptoms that persist for many years after the injury. Cognitive symptoms have been found to be linked to reduced productivity in work and it is generally recommended to use early intervention to reduce the longer-term impact of cognitive symptoms and facilitate participation in social activity.

If ongoing symptoms are thought to be psychological, then it is reasonable for treatment to be psychological therapy. However, what about the somatic/physical symptoms and cognitive symptoms? Is a talking therapy alone going to tackle them and if not, who and what else needs to be involved?

In the following chapter we detail the different types of professionals that can provide assessment and treatment for the range of symptoms individuals experience after an mTBI.

6

Where to seek help: professional roles and responsibilities

Accident and Emergency (A&E)

Not all people who suffer a head injury are taken or take themselves to A&E straight away, especially if they fall into the subgroup where they do not experience symptoms immediately and are more than likely in shock. Lots of my clients have told me that they did not want to 'make a fuss' or just wanted to get home, which is an automatic need of the nervous system to seek safety. Some individuals have told me that other people that witnessed the injury offered to call them an ambulance or to be taken to hospital, but they declined at the time.

If they do attend A&E, experiences can be highly variable and unfortunately there is not a standardized level of service and care across different hospitals. Some individuals receive a CT scan to check for any structural issues or internal bleeding, but more often than not, the CT is reassuringly clear, and people are sent on their way with a leaflet on head injury/ concussion and told to look out for any worrying symptoms. I have had clients that have asked their A&E doctor what they should and shouldn't do when they get home; many are told they do not need to make any changes, and some are told to take cognitive rest.

There are a proportion of individuals that attend A&E a few days later as symptoms start to develop. Again, the experience is variable, but is mostly one of undergoing simple investigations such as blood tests and observations. When no major issues are found, they are given medical reassurance that the investigations are normal. I really empathize with stretched services in A&E departments given that this injury does not present as a classic emergency and there is a high chance that presenting symptoms will resolve. The number of patients that are referred for a clinical head injury follow up is minimal. If they are fortunate enough to be seen as an outpatient as a follow up, they are often discharged after the appointment with no further treatment due to the lack of specialist services available.

General practitioner (GP)

For those individuals that do not attend an emergency hospital setting after their injury, the majority do visit their GP; this can often be the first point of contact with a medical professional. GPs are amazing in knowing a little about a lot of medical health conditions and as such, are usually the point of referral onto other specialists.

There has been some research exploring GPs' knowledge and approach to concussions and its diagnosis. The findings reveal that knowledge and management practice is varied especially when comparing GPs in different locations (e.g. urban vs more rural). Given that GPs see individuals with acute concussion as well as those with prolonged and persistent symptoms after a head injury, identifying, diagnosis and referring on for targeted treatment is likely to improve outcomes for individuals. This will then decrease socio-economic and health burden.

As such, GPs play an important role in the acute phase of symptom management after a head injury therefor the need for ongoing concussion education and awareness is essential for primary care providers so that key features are not overlooked and treatment can be started early.

Box 5. Anna describes her experience with her GP

Two days after my car accident I went to see a walk-in GP who told me to use Ibuprofen gel on my shoulder. At that point I was only aware of intense physical pain, not neurological symptoms. Following this, I started noticing symptoms such as dizziness and feeling off balance, distorted vision and cognitive issues like forgetfulness and slower processing. After a few days, I went to see my GP who diagnosed me with concussion. Regarding my vision, he said my prescription was probably out of date and suggested I book an optician's appointment. He also gave me a business card for the local NHS physiotherapy service, prescribed strong painkillers and organized some blood tests for me which came back showing low vitamin D levels.

Neurology

A neurologist is a medically trained doctor that specializes in diagnosis and managing and treating disorders of the brain and nervous system. These include stroke, Parkinson's disease, epilepsy, dementia such as Alzheimer's disease, multiple sclerosis and other more rare neurological diseases and conditions. Given that a concussion is an insult to the brain and nervous system, neurologists are the medical specialists that diagnose the presence and severity of a brain injury. As well as conducting a neurological examination themselves which can include basic 'bedside' cognitive testing as well assessment of motor skills, reflexes and sensory functions; these doctors usually send for additional tests and investigations such as brain scans, blood tests, detailed cognitive assessment as well as genetic testing. They then collate all the detailed information from a variety of sources to assist them in their differential diagnosis.

It is actually quite uncommon for someone with a concussion to see a neurologist unless they have persistent neurological symptoms such as headaches, issues with memory, dizziness, sleep disturbance and chronic pain. In terms of a neurologist role, they may send you for more specific, non-routine investigations like an MRI, or nerve conduction studies. They may prescribe medication for headaches or refer someone on for specialist intervention. For example, if they find that someone is suffering with dizziness, they may refer on for vestibular rehabilitation, or if they identify issues with visual tracking, they will refer on for vision therapy. Both of these specialists will be discussed below.

Box 6. Anna details her experiences of neurology services over a period of two years after her injury

Approximately eight months after my injury, an appointment came through to see a neurologist at my local hospital. He got me to do a few exercises and checked my balance and reflexes. He then gave me a short cognitive test for people with dementia. I answered all the questions correctly apart from one where I had to read a simple sentence then remember it and write it down. I missed out part of the sentence which I was surprised at because I had previously had a pretty photographic memory and I was certain that pre-injury I would have remembered it exactly as it was.

An MRI scan of my brain was arranged, which came back showing a small bleed. The neurologist didn't think this was caused by the car accident and said I could have had it since childhood. I don't know what to think about that and I guess I'll never know the answer. He diagnosed me with non-organic post-concussion syndrome with functional symptoms. He referred me to a neuro-physiotherapist to help me with my dizziness and balance issues (the treatment for this was very effective and I write about it later under the 'Physiotherapy' section of this book.) He also recommended the medication Gabapentin for my anxiety.

My husband accompanied me to a second appointment with the neurologist a few months later. He'd arranged for me to have a CT scan which came back normal. He could see that I was still struggling with symptoms and referred me to a local brain injury clinic. I was pleased about the referral but, in the end, I didn't attend as

---

my first appointment four months later coincided with my neuropsy-chological treatment with Dr Pradhan. As well as not wishing to duplicate treatment, I'd have had to travel over 25 miles to the clinic for appointments, and at the time I couldn't drive and long-distance travel triggered my symptoms. I rang the clinic to say that I had alter-native treatment, and the lady I spoke to told me that people with 'mild' brain injuries often 'slip through the net' which is why it can be so hard and take so long to find appropriate treatment.

Two years after my injury, another neurologist, with expertise in mild traumatic brain injury diagnosed me with a concussion/diffuse axonal injury caused by the acceleration/deceleration of the forces of the car accident causing my brain to bounce around inside my skull. By this point I'd had quite a lot of different treatments and had done a lot of my own recovery interventions. I'd improved a lot but not fully. The neurologist told me that as I was two years post-injury, it was likely that I'd plateaued in my recovery, but he encouraged me to keep going with whatever was helping. I remember feeling relieved to receive the diagnosis but I was also scared of the impli-cations of not making a full recovery.

Neuro-optometry

An injury to the head can result in an interruption in commu-nication between the eyes and the brain, which can cause a whole host of symptoms including blurred vision, sensitivity to light, reading difficulty, headaches when doing physical tasks, reduction or loss of visual field, and difficulties with eye movements. It is often the case that visual function is overlooked in diagnosing brain injury symptoms, particularly during initial assessment and treatment of the injury. As you will recall, Anna's GP had never heard of a concussion causing visual issues and suggested that she get her eyes tested. However, this is not an issue solely with the eyes, but rather with the way that the eyes and the brain are able to interact. Treatment of vision problems after a concussion can have a major and positive impact on outcome and as such, if someone is experiencing visual symptoms after a head injury they can benefit from a neuro-optometric assessment and treatment plan.

A neuro-optometric rehabilitation optometrist is an eye care professional who specializes in the diagnosis and rehabilitation of visual, perceptual, and motor disorders. Increased research in this field is documenting the improved performance of people who have completed a vision rehabilitation program after a concussion. Neuro-optometric therapy includes, but is not limited to, acquired strabismus, diplopia, binocular dysfunction, convergence and/or accommodation paresis/paralysis, oculomotor dysfunction, visual-spatial dysfunction, visual perceptual and cognitive deficits, and traumatic visual acuity loss.

Often visual dysfunctions can manifest themselves as psychological outcomes such as anxiety and panic disorders as well as spatial dysfunctions affecting balance and posture. A neuro-optometric rehabilitation treatment plan can improve vision dysfunction as a result of a head injury. Some of the treatment methods include non-compensatory lenses and prisms with and without occlusion as well as other appropriate medical rehabilitation strategies.

As well as visual problems being overlooked during initial treatment of a brain injury and PCS, symptoms may not reveal themselves for some time following the injury. If you notice any changes in your vision following a concussion or some other head trauma, the advice is not to ignore them. First port of call is your GP who can then hopefully refer you on to a specialist to help determine the cause of the vision change. Early diagnosis leads to appropriate treatment such as a Neuro-optometric rehabilitation optometrist. Left untreated, visual system disorders can have serious consequences for day-to-day function, fatigue levels and confidence in interacting with the world. This is due to the person's inability to organize and make sense of visual information, the presence of poor depth perception and difficulties concerning posture, which can then contribute to secondary pain.

Vision also plays a significant role in someone's ability to balance, orient themselves in space, and process movement of things in their environment. Approximately 20 per cent of the nerve fibres from the eye neural tracts (the neural fibres within the brain that connect to the eye) interact with the vestibular system, the parts of the inner ear and brain that help control balance and eye movements. Balance is also supported by sensory information received through joints and muscles.

Box 7. Anna details her experience of neuro-optometry input

A couple of months after my injury, an optometrist checked my eyesight, and my prescription was the same as pre-accident. However, I was still having problems with focusing and reading. As an avid reader, not being able to read properly for any length of time really upset me, especially as I wasn't able to properly read bedtime stories to my children. I was given a coloured overlay to put over written text, which calmed everything down and stopped the words jumping around. I later bought some glasses with pink-tinted lenses which I used for reading text in books and on screens. Both of these helped me to focus for longer stretches of time. I was able to read more, write, use a computer for longer and look at screens more comfortably. I also wore the glasses sometimes when I went out in the sun or to a place with bright artificial lights. Eventually, I no longer needed the tinted overlays and glasses.

Audio-vestibular physicians

The auditory system is responsible for the sense of hearing and consists of the outer ear, middle ear, cochlea (and its nerves and nuclei), limbic system, auditory and attention pathways.

The vestibular system includes the inner ear and brain. It integrates the vestibular, visual, proprioceptive and auditory inputs as well as gravity receptors and feedback circuits. These are then processed by the body to assist balance and enable eye movements, muscle activity and autonomic (unconscious) responses.

The vestibular system is susceptible to damage when the head and upper body is subjected to injury. The result is that people may experience difficulty with balance and movement, as well as with their perception of space, which has an impact on all aspects of their day-to-day life. Human balance is sensed by three peripheral sensors: the vestibular system, the ophthalmological system and the proprioceptive system. Symptoms can be more pronounced when put in environments with excessive visual stimulation, such as supermarkets with strip lighting, or dark roads with bright headlights of oncoming traffic.

Audio-vestibular physicians undertake investigations, diagnosis and management of the medical aspect of disorders of hearing, balance and tinnitus. While the focus of audio-vestibular medicine may seem like a narrow focus, the specialty covers multiple systems and disorders such as dizziness, hearing loss, tinnitus, imbalance, eye movement disorders and speech problems of peripheral otological and central nervous system origin. The specialty covers all age ranges and has a strong interest in rehabilitation, including the management of the social and psychological impact of these disorders. It is a specialty that can make a significant difference to an individual's quality of life and can be found in a variety of settings from community-based clinics through to highly specialist academic centres.

Physiotherapy

As with other allied professionals, there are a few branches of speciality within physiotherapy. Musculoskeletal (MSK) Physiotherapists focus on the body's bones, muscles, cartilage, tendons, ligaments, joints and other connective tissues which all carry out vital roles such as supporting the body, allowing movement and protecting delicate internal organs. Often people that suffer from mTBI have whiplash and soft tissue injuries and working with a MSK physiotherapist can help reduce inflammation and promote body-based healing. MSK physiotherapists tend to use a variety of tools and treatments including manual therapy and the use of hands-on techniques (e.g. massage, stretching, manipulation) to help with mobilization and improvement of function. They also develop and provide exercise programmes for clients to use outside of the treatment sessions to facilitate greatest efficacy of the hands-on treatment.

Neuro-physiotherapists predominantly work with individuals diagnosed with neurological conditions, particularly those that have suffered strokes or are diagnosed with neurological movement disorders such as Parkinson's disease. The neuro-physiotherapist's role is to help those with neurological conditions either progress in neurorehabilitation or to reduce the impact of the neurological condition on their physical function and, ultimately, quality of life. Some neuro-physiotherapists also have specialist knowledge and training in treating vestibular disorders which is very relevant for those with mTBI and PCS.

Box 8. Anna details her experience of physiotherapy treatment

From about ten days after my car accident, I had regular appointments with a physiotherapist at my house for several weeks. She gave me manual therapy, acupuncture and various exercises to promote movement in my back, arm, neck and head and recommended a gentle Pilates DVD. I subsequently saw an NHS physiotherapist who helped me to gain mobility in my torso and walk properly again. The physiotherapy helped me a lot, especially to gain some of my physical functioning but unfortunately it didn't fully remove my pain and it didn't really address my concussion directly, even though I did learn about the nervous system.

I had some big breakthroughs about a year post-injury when I saw a neuro-physiotherapist at my local hospital via referral from the NHS neurologist. I think over the next few months I saw her two or three times. She treated me for Benign Paroxysmal Positional Vertigo (BPPV), which is when tiny crystals get dislodged in the inner ear, which happened when I had my accident. To treat this, she explained the condition to me and then, with another physiotherapist, performed the Epley Manoeuvre on me a couple of times each at two different appointments. This involved being laid back on a bed and having my head tipped over the edge and moved to the side in a particular way to dislodge the particles and help them to settle back to where they should be. I had to take it easy for a while afterwards.

She also gave me gaze stabilization exercises, balance exercises and spoke to me about vestibular migraines. For these she recommended 400 mg daily of vitamin B2 (riboflavin) as recommended by Professor Owen Judd on the website <www.vestibularmigraine. co.uk>. All this treatment went a long way to resolving my dizziness and balance problems.

The gaze stabilization exercises also helped to correct my vision issues. For these, I had to stare at a fixed point on a wall and move my head from side to side, keeping my gaze on the point, for about a minute at a time. I did this several times a day and built up to several minutes at a time and gradually, as my dizziness subsided, my eyes were able to focus much better.

Endocrinology

Endocrinology is a specialty service that sees people with a range of hormonal diseases. For many people their problems occur because they either produce too much or have too little of a particular hormone. Deficiency of a hormone can cause symptoms that are difficult to diagnose and that can make people feel unwell in peculiar ways.

Post traumatic endocrine dysfunction is a well-recognized complication of traumatic brain injury, but less attention is paid to it than to concussion and mTBI. Dr Mark L Gordon is an interventional endocrinologist and world leader in this field of specialist treatment, and via his research has found that TBI can not only cause physical, cognitive, emotional and behavioural symptoms, but can also cause, or accelerate, hormonal deficiencies or insufficiencies which can also lead to physical, physiological and psychological problems. At least 50 per cent of people with a TBI showed some loss of pituitary hormone function immediately after the brain injury occurred. The pituitary gland is sometimes called the 'master gland' of the endocrine system because it controls the functions of many of the other endocrine glands. The pituitary gland is no larger than a pea and is located at the base of the brain. The gland is attached to the hypothalamus (a part of the brain that affects the pituitary gland) by nerve fibres and blood vessels. Around 50 per cent of people develop new pituitary hormone deficiencies a year after the injury. This leads to a reduction in regulation of the thyroid gland, the adrenal glands and the male reproductive organs, which are all vital in the production of critical hormones in the body.

Many people with TBI may have endocrine defects and, more significantly, a growth hormone deficiency which can lead to reduced energy and feelings of lethargy, even if things look normal on examination. GPs may refer to a consultant endocrinologist to conduct a full assessment of pituitary function, which can start with baseline blood tests and also include an insulin tolerance test to look for growth hormone deficiency.

Neuropsychiatry

Neuropsychiatrists are trained as medical doctors who then go on to specialize in psychiatry and then neuropsychiatry. They are trained in, and have expertise in dealing with, mental disorders that are connected to the brain and nervous system. They can be seen as the bridge between neurology and psychiatry.

Neuropsychiatrists mainly work with patients who have psychiatric illnesses (e.g. depression, anxiety disorder, psychosis) that originate from a neurological injury or disorder, for example epilepsy, TBI, stroke, Parkinson's disease and FND. It is a growing specialty and neuropsychiatrists work in a variety of settings and services and are often embedded in multidisciplinary teams.

A neuropsychiatrist has many skills in terms of diagnosing and making treatment plans as well as being a specialist in prescribing medications for psychiatric disorders that arise in the context of a brain pathology. With an mTBI, a neuropsychiatrist can prescribe medication to help those experiencing significant anxiety and depression, as well as sleep disturbance and fatigue. Often by treating these symptoms, the individual is better able to focus on their recovery. Generally, people gain most benefit from prescribed medications when they are combined with neuropsychological intervention.

Clinical neuropsychology

A clinical neuropsychologist is someone who has completed a doctoral level of training in clinical psychology but then goes on to do further specialized training in the field of neuropsychology. Like neuropsychiatrists, neuropsychologists predominantly work with people who have neurological conditions or diagnoses. Although they have an understanding of medication, they are not medical doctors and don't have the qualification or knowledge to prescribe. Clinically, neuropsychologists focus on assessment and treatment.

In terms of assessment, the clinical neuropsychologist gathers information from a variety of sources to develop a 'formulation'. A formulation is a process whereby different pieces of information about the individual, their experiences, beliefs, life story, physical, emotional and cognitive functioning are understood in terms of their relationship and interaction with each other and with the issues they present (i.e. neurological condition). A neuropsychologist might help neurologists and neuropsychiatrists in the differential diagnosis of presenting symptoms by using standardized cognitive tests and interpreting the results in the context of the person's case history, symptoms, and what family and friends are reporting. For example, are the memory problems that someone is describing due to changes in the brain (such as dementia) or are they caused by a mental disorder (such as depression)? Usually the answer is a complex interaction of what is referred to as organic (physical) and non-organic (psychological).

For mTBI, traditional neuropsychological tests were developed to assess deficits in mainly cortical functions (e.g. language, memory, visuo-spatial functions) and in neurodegenerative conditions (Alzheimer's disease). Because of this, it is possible that many standard neuropsychological tests are not fit for purpose for injuries and conditions that are more subcortical in nature (i.e. PCS).

In many cases, neuropsychological testing reveals only subtle and relative weakness in processing speed, attention, memory and areas of executive function. Depending on how the clinician interprets them, the test scores may come back as 'unremarkable' as they are not statistically below what is considered the 'normal range' of performance.

There are many different neuropsychological tests available. In my clinic, we use a mix of tests that assess general intellectual functioning, focal tests that tap into more cortical functions as well as more contemporary tests that tap into high-order processing speed and attention. This allows us to gather information on cognitive functions that are affected and those that may be unaffected or spared; we build a profile of cognitive strengths and weaknesses and use it to tailor cognitive strategies and rehabilitation.

On the whole, people apply themselves the best they can during the assessment, which can be a challenging experience. Many report that they were completely 'wiped out' afterwards. In terms of the findings, a large percentage of individuals have a profile showing reduced function (sometimes very subtle) in the subcortical/white matter pathways. This is usually against the backdrop of a normal performance across a range of more traditional tests that assess intellect and cortical cognitive functions.

Of course, there are differences between the 'sterile' testing environment (i.e. a clinic room) and a real-world setting. The neuropsychological assessment is conducted on a one-to-one basis, in a structured manner, with all efforts made to minimize distractions (e.g. noise, phones, other people). The reason for this approach is to ensure the validity, reliability and standardization of the assessment and subsequent results. The aim of a neuropsychology cognitive assessment is to obtain objective information that should only be affected by cognitive status (as much as realistically possible), as opposed to any other distractions in the environment. The disadvantage of this approach, which has been argued to lack 'ecological validity', is that the testing environment can help clients compensate for subtle cognitive difficulties, due to the imposed structure and limitation of distraction.

Within a real-world setting, be that at home, in a work situation or social situation, there are numerous cognitive and psychological demands. The presence of distractions and time pressures, along with the impact of fatigue, can magnify even subtle cognitive problems, which can then prove to be very debilitating, especially in a work context. Often clients rely heavily on external compensatory strategies, particularly at work, such as writing everything down, which is usually a strategy that was not required before the injury. Many clients report they were able to hold a lot more information in mind and routinely multi-task prior to their injury. They also have to curb other activities (e.g. socializing, being active in family life, hobbies) so that they have the energy levels to function at work.

It is quite challenging to capture behavioural and emotional self-regulation, associated with frontal and subcortical pathways in the brain, during a neuropsychological assessment. These pathways affect individuals' ability to integrate the motivational, reward/risk, emotional and social aspects of behaviours. This can't be assessed with standard neuropsychological tests but instead is usually assessed by how an individual functions in their everyday life. Post-injury, are they able to integrate what is needed in stressful social situations and respond in a way that is metered and rational? What do clients' family members describe in terms of changes they observe in their loved ones? Some people observe their family members to be less empathic, be more egocentric, have a tendency to lose their temper quickly and take things the wrong way following the injury. Many clients describe themselves to be snappier and more irritable and have a desire to socially withdraw.

In terms of treatment and intervention, a neuropsychologist may draw upon a range of approaches and tools from their clinical psychology training and knowledge of neurorehabilitation to help individuals and families following a neurological event or diagnosis. The importance of being treated by a neuropsychologist versus a psychologist that does not have expertise or knowledge of brain and nervous system disorders is that the origin of symptoms someone presents with may be misunderstood. For example, the feelings of anxiety and panic that someone experiences in the context of TBI are not solely cognitive in nature, they are usually first and foremost due to the dysregulation of the nervous system (as a result of neuro-trauma) and also contributed to by reduced cognitive capacity and a lower threshold for dealing with external sensory input (e.g. noise, bright lights). When someone's system gets overloaded, the brain and body try to close down as a protective mechanism. This can result in negative cognitive appraisals ('what is happening to me, what is wrong with me, why can't I cope?') and leads to avoidance of similar situations. A therapist without neuro experience may try to modify the beliefs first before helping to regulate the person's nervous system. This could be futile as the origin of their panic is not cognitive but physical, so intervention needs to start with helping the individual move into parasympathetic mode so that they are more resourced to deal with sensory overload and cognitive inefficiencies. After someone is in a more grounded place and understands why this cycle is happening, only then can they move into focusing on negative cognitive appraisals of their situation and make a subsequent behavioural change.

It is important for you, the reader, to be aware that the focus of neuropsychological treatment for those that have persistent symptoms following an mTBI is not necessarily about full recovery. It is about developing strategies and acceptance of the chronic and persisting symptoms that are associated with a small percentage of mTBI clients, as well as developing psychological resilience, adaptation and self-compassion. Post-TBI fatigue can be a lifelong challenge and you may have to make daily choices about what activities you partake in and how you 'spend' your energy in order to successfully manage the impact of fatigue on your symptom presentation and day-to-day functioning. You will have to weigh up the pros and cons, and balance dealing with ongoing challenges, especially fatigue, and your quality of life. For example, you may need to choose whether you put all your energy into work or reduce work so that you can allocate some of your energy to social activities and family time. Before a brain injury, this was not a choice you would have had to make – you would have had the resources to do both.

> **Box 9. Anna details her experiences of neuropsychological assessment and treatment**
>
> In December 2017, about a year after my accident, I underwent neuropsychological testing with Dr Pradhan. My test results showed that I was borderline impaired in a number of areas where previously I would have likely performed at an above-average level. That was devastating to hear on the one hand and, on the other, it was strangely reassuring to know that the challenges I was experiencing were measurable and not imaginary. In spite of the low test scores, I knew I'd already made progress since my accident so I was hopeful there were more improvements to come.
>
> In June 2018, I had further neuropsychological testing with Dr Pradhan. My results showed that I'd improved in a number of areas, and some of my scores had gone from borderline impaired to average. I was thrilled.
>
> I subsequently had a number of individual therapy sessions with Dr Pradhan which really helped me on a cognitive, emotional, physical, psychological and spiritual level. She helped me to understand my brain and nervous system and provided me with education, strategies and techniques to help me both come to terms with my situation and also recover further, which was very empowering.
>
> Dr Pradhan recommended I do a regular movement practice and she found one for me she thought I'd enjoy called 'Movingness', which combined breathing, dance, meditation and mindfulness. For the first time in over a year, I could do exercise without sending my nervous system into overdrive.

Neuro occupational therapy

The aim and purpose of occupational therapy is to enable clients to manage their day-to-day tasks and activities in a way that contributes to their physical, social and emotional well-being while accounting for and adapting to their limitations, be that physical, cognitive, emotional, behavioural or a combination of them all. The main focus of occupational therapy is rehabilitation.

An occupational therapist will work with you to address dysfunction using interventions that may look at altering the way a task is performed, adapting the physical environment, teaching you a new skill or working with you to regain old ones.

A comprehensive initial assessment by the occupational therapist should cover areas such as:

- past and current medical history
- current impairments and how these impact on daily activities
- goals (short-term and long-term) that the client and family have
- a physical functional assessment and also if indicated a cognitive screening test.

An occupational therapist with a neuro specialism assesses the whole person and is equipped to understand the challenges faced by those with neurological impairments and have the unique skill of creating individualized solutions for people.

Box 10. Anna details her experience of working with occupational therapists

I was fortunate to have support from two neuro occupational therapists, one of whom was from my local branch of Headway, the UK brain injury charity. I've included some of their recommendations in the chapter, 'Cognitive Rest Versus Cognitive Strategies'.

The occupational therapists helped me to plan my days and weeks, learn how to manage my fatigue levels, pace myself and implement strategies to make life simpler and smoother.

I'm grateful for all the help I had from them because I was able to gradually build up my energy levels, do more things around the house, drive more, organize my life more effectively, look after my family better and sleep better. I learned to focus on what I could do and not be overly concerned with what I couldn't do, knowing that if I kept trying and kept working on things, they'd improve.

Speech and language therapy

Speech and Language Therapists (SLTs) have a range of skills and training and work with a variety of people who have difficulty with verbally expressing themselves, communicating and understanding others. SLTs often work with people that suffer with swallowing or eating problems after neurological conditions such as stroke. Some people, after having a mTBI, have difficulty with finding the right words, expressing themselves coherently and picking up nuances in what other people are saying. An SLT can work with that person to improve these issues and they often work jointly with neuropsychologists. For example, if someone is having issues with word finding, it may cause anticipatory anxiety in situations where they have experienced this difficulty before (like social events or work meetings). Unfortunately, this pre-empting of a situational challenge usually results in the difficulty being more pronounced and individuals may find themselves wanting to avoid such situations. Using the tools provided by SLT along with psychological strategies can assist a person to manage these issues.

SLT can usually be accessed via a referral from your doctor or consultant. In the UK, you can also self-refer to your local speech and language therapy service. Alternatively, you can arrange to see a therapist privately.

Specialist nutrition (dietician)

This is a growing area of specialism in the field of neuro-rehab. Dieticians can work across the spectrum of severity of neurological disorders and conditions and can assess to see if people are getting the right nutrition to optimize their recovery. This can range from education on the best foods to help improve fatigue and avoid boom and busts in energy levels, managing changes in digestion and gut issues post-injury, to how to achieve and maintain a healthy weight. By getting the fundamentals around nutrition and hydration right from the start, people can get the most out of other aspects of specialist input and rehab. Given there is such a wealth of information available at our fingertips and some of it can be conflicting, having an expert to guide you through this minefield and collaborate with other clinicians you have involved in your rehab, can be really beneficial.

Anna has done a lot of research into different supplements as she did not have access to a specialist dietician. Information she has gathered can be found in Chapter 8.

Multidisciplinary neurorehabilitation

Recovery from a brain injury can really vary from individual to individual and an essential part of the rehabilitation process is balancing hope with realism. It is vital that rehab therapists are open about what to expect in terms of the level of recovery and what factors can optimize this.

For all clinicians working in this field, neurorehabilitation is a two-way process and success of which depends largely on two things:

1 The skill of the therapist/clinician in finding out what is important to the client in order to be able to set goals that are meaningful and rehab around this.
2 The client's readiness to engage in therapy at that specific time, because they want to recover and have the motivation to do so.

Clinicians who work in the field of neurorehabilitation aim to work together to achieve the best possible outcome for the client and their family. There is overlap between all the disciplines. Collaborative working is vital for cohesion and consistency for the client. Clinicians may provide input all at the same time during the course of someone's recovery journey, which has its advantages and disadvantages. An advantage of this approach is that it provides a holistic package of rehabilitation where goals are client-focused rather than discipline-focused. For example, the client's goal may be to return to work, which would require an OT who specializes in vocational rehabilitation and can assist with cognitive strategies and fatigue management, physiotherapy to assist with strength and stamina and neuropsychology to provide information that guides the cognitive strategies and provide support and strategies with regard to emotional regulation and adjustment. However, sometimes a multidisciplinary approach can feel quite overwhelming for the client as they feel they have lots of appointments to manage from different clinicians. To try and combat this scheduling burden, I often suggest the clinicians provide joint sessions where possible. Joint sessions are very beneficial for helping people achieve goals that fall across a number of disciplines and they also avoid duplication or confliction.

Integrative medicine and functional medicine

Integrative medicine is a holistic medical discipline which takes into account the lifestyle habits of an individual. The physician works to treat the whole person rather than just the disease. As such, the physician considers the mind, body and soul of a patient when looking at ways to promote healing and well-being.

Integrative medicine not only uses a combination of modern healthcare practices to diagnose and treat a person but also draws upon other 'alternative' treatment modalities such as acupuncture, yoga, or massage. Integrative medicine physicians believe that lifestyle choices are the root cause of many modern chronic diseases and so focus on nutritional and exercise habits of the individual to target the whole host of issues that can be related to obesity and diabetes.

Similarly, functional medicine practitioners seek to work closely with the individual to get to the root cause of health problems, rather than just addressing the symptoms. They view the different functions of the body as an integrated system rather than separate systems. They carry out lab tests, in-depth interviews with the patient and seek to uncover and treat underlying and chronic health conditions.

Although integrative medicine and functional medicine have similarities, in that they focus on supporting the patient as a whole person, functional medicine strives to determine the root cause of each and every disease, particularly chronic diseases such as autoimmune and cardiovascular diseases, as well as diabetes and obesity. Rather than simply making a diagnosis and then determining which drugs or surgery will best treat the condition, functional medicine practitioners dive deep into the patient's history and biochemistry to ask 'why is this patient ill?' Functional medicine is highly personalized and often includes a detailed analysis of an individual's genetic makeup.

Latest advances in medical science are supporting a move towards personalized medicine and new technology is allowing for individualized testing. For example specialized clinics in North America and other parts of the world are offering a range of individualized testing such as genomics (genetics testing), metabolomics (testing individual biochemistry), microbion studies (to identify imbalances in gut organisms which can impact on health) as well as autonomics assessments, which can explore the balance between the 'fight/flight' and 'rest/ digest' branches of the autonomic nervous system, as this has been found to be an issue in chronic conditions. Many clinicians are seeing personalized medicine being the future model of medical care.

Legal input

A proportion, around half of my clients at any one time, are involved, or have been involved, in litigation. That is, pursuing a personal injury claim for compensation for their injuries from an event or incident that was not their fault and the subsequent impact on their lives. While overall the experiences can differ from person to person, an overriding theme is how stressful it can be for individuals and families to go through this process. However, getting the right legal team can actually help fund the investigations and treatments that are not readily available via statutory health services. Given ever-increasing wait times in an underfunded and under-resourced health service, being able to access rehabilitation early (albeit in the private sector) can be life changing due to the positive impact it can have on outcome and prognosis for the individual. For many people, however, this is not an option if their injury occurred in a situation where there is no liability and no insurance cover. These individuals are left on long waiting lists or have to seek out and fund services themselves.

Box 11. Anna details her experience and thoughts of the legal system

I want to include a quick note here on pursuing a personal injury claim for compensation, if that's relevant to you. If you've been injured by someone else and you're eligible to make a claim, then I recommend that you find a solicitor specializing in concussion/mild brain injury cases. Mild brain injury cases are complex, and the legal system is complicated to navigate, especially if you've had a head injury. A good specialist solicitor will help you to access expert medical help and on-going support in a timely manner, can arrange for interim payments as your case proceeds, will support you as you navigate the legal system and will negotiate the best financial outcome for you. You may have had to take time off work, changed jobs and/or incurred considerable expense during your recovery and suffered in other ways as a result of your injury. Compensation will not solve all your problems, but it can go some way to redressing your situation and can help provide the best possible path to recovery, security and peace of mind.

7

Adjunct therapies, methods and treatment tools

As each person's constellation of symptoms associated with PCS can vary, there is no one set pathway of recovery. Many people benefit from a multi-faceted approach to their recovery and often combine a number of treatments and therapies. Different treatments will help different people, depending on the individual, their injury and symptoms, and what resonates with them, which can, of course, change over time. Another factor is treatment availability, not only in terms of location but also financial viability. Some people can find specialized healthcare providers nearby but others end up travelling long distances, including to other countries, to find specialist treatment. However, with the increase in access to video calling platforms (Skype, Zoom, Microsoft Teams) it is possible for some treatments to take place remotely which opens one up to a world of options.

Below is a list of different holistic treatments and therapies with a very brief description, covering many different facets and stages of recovery. This list has been collated via a combination of my clinical knowledge and Anna's personal experiences, research and discussions with other people with concussion. Some of them are considered to be 'alternative' therapies, and some of them are more known in the US than in the UK. They are not exclusively modalities for PCS, and they are not in and of themselves cures, but they may assist you in your recovery. They may be suitable to pursue alongside or after some of the other more first-line treatments and modalities mentioned in this book.

If any of these approaches appeal to you, then explore them further and see if there is a provider near you or online. If you decide to try a therapy or treatment, make sure the practitioner is qualified in their field, and while not compulsory, it is more beneficial if the therapist has had experience of treating concussion/mTBIs. If that is not possible, then try to find a therapist who is sympathetic and understanding of your health issues. Inform your doctor or involved clinicians of any alternative or holistic treatments you are undergoing and check with them that it is a suitable treatment for your situation and ensure that there are no contraindications. While this list is comprehensive, it is not exhaustive, there are many other alternative treatments that are available.

Osteopathy

Osteopathy uses physical manipulation, stretching and massage and is based on the principle that the well-being of an individual depends on their bones, muscles, ligaments and connective tissue functioning smoothly together. Osteopaths can help increase the mobility of joints, relieve muscle tension, reduce pain, enhance blood supply to tissues and help the body to heal. As such, people often go and see an osteopath if they have back pain, neck pain, shoulder pain, arthritis, hip and pelvic issues as well as sports injury. Given that osteopathy tends to focus on general manual therapy techniques, there can be some overlap with physiotherapists and chiropractors. Most osteopaths work privately as there is limited funding available within the NHS. To an osteopath, for your body to work well, its structure must also work well, so osteopaths work to restore your body to a state of balance where possible, without the use of drugs or surgery. Osteopaths also advise on posture and exercise to aid recovery, promote health and prevent symptoms recurring.

Box 12. Anna sought the input of an osteopath and describes her experience

I worked with an osteopath for several weeks. As well as giving me manual therapy and acupuncture, he taught me the importance of exercise and lifestyle, and explained the link between stress and emotions, pain, diet, sleep, and so on. While this didn't cure the pain, it significantly reduced it and ever since I've been able to manage it much better. Over a couple of months, I went from walking with a stick to riding a bike for the first time in two years and regularly swimming 20 lengths.

Chiropractic neurology

Registered practitioners of chiropractic neurology have a deep understanding of the brain and nervous system and can treat many of the symptoms of concussion such as dizziness, headaches, vision issues as well as musculoskeletal problems. They can also advise on creating a sustainable healthy and balanced lifestyle. In the US, these health professionals are sometimes called 'functional neurologists'. This is different from a functional neurologist in the UK, who treats people with functional neurological disorder (FND).

Eye movement desensitisation reprocessing (EMDR)

EMDR is a psychotherapy treatment that helps people process distressing memories by using eye movements. EMDR has been extensively researched and proven effective to help people who are experiencing trauma, including PTSD and the problems that trauma can result in like flashbacks, upsetting thoughts or images, hypervigilance, anxiety and low mood. In the first stage, the therapist gathers information about an individual's current situation, their life (including relationships) and distressing events in order to discuss possible targets for EMDR processing and developing a treatment plan. The therapist then works on creating a safe place before the processing part of the intervention commences. There has been a substantial increase in EMDR training programmes and more and more clinical psychologists and psychotherapists are undertaking training in EMDR to add to their 'therapeutic tool bag'. What is unique about EMDR is that the individual does not need to verbally go over their traumatic experiences and memories in depth with the therapist at each session, but rather they are supported to bring them to mind while the processing occurs.

A proportion of my clients with a mTBI have undergone EMDR prior to our sessions starting. The focus of the EMDR can be processing the traumatic memories they may have associated with the injury or aftermath, or there may be more long-term traumatic memories that have never been processed properly but are reactivated in the context of the mTBI. I have found that when individuals have partaken in some trauma-focused work, they are then better equipped to make use of cognitive strategies and behavioural activation without being side-tracked by emotional triggers.

Brainspotting

Brainspotting is a relatively newly developed treatment method that works by identifying, processing and releasing core neurophysiological sources of emotional/body pain, trauma dissociation and a variety of other symptoms that can be challenging to live with.

A 'brainspot' is a point in visual space that a client has a strong reaction to. Developed by David Grant PhD, he found that where you look is associated with how you feel and this is connected to the deeper, subcortical part of the brain. The therapist will ask the client to look at different spots in their visual field and communicate how they are feeling, the therapist also simultaneously is on the lookout for non-verbal information arising in the client's body that can give clues to their emotional status.

Not only can this therapy help with symptoms of anxiety, depression and trauma, it can also help with issues that are holding people back, and some say it allows them to tap into areas of suppressed creativity. The late Robert Scaer in his book 'The Trauma Spectrum' details how brainspotting is not just about activating the parasympathetic nervous system, it is also about bringing homeostasis in the nervous system.

Somatic experiencing (SE)

SE was created by Dr Peter Levine, PhD, an expert in the field of trauma whose experience of being knocked over by a pedestrian is detailed in Chapter 2. This therapy works on the principle that trauma gets trapped in the body, leading to some of the symptoms people with PTSD or people who have experienced trauma might experience. Using this method, practitioners work on releasing this stress from the body through a framework known as SIBAM (Sensation, Imagery, Behaviour, Affect and Meaning). SE helps individuals have an increased sense of awareness of their internal experience (interoceptive, proprioceptive and kinesthetic sensations) which then provides a platform to help with emotional regulation. essentially, while most talking therapies such as CBT use 'top down' methods (looking at thoughts and cognition first), Somatic experiencing uses a 'bottom up' approach, which starts with bodily sensations before moving onto thoughts.

There are many therapists who may refer to their work as somatic but somatic experiencing therapy is a particular method developed by Dr Levine and you can find a list of qualified practitioners on the following website: <https://directory. traumahealing.org/>

Trauma release exercises (TRE)

TRE are a series of physical exercises designed to help release deeply stored stress, trauma and tension from the body and calm the nervous system. They were developed by David Berceli, PhD, originally to treat people with PTSD in conflict zones. You can find some of the exercises on YouTube, in books and on apps for a self-help approach but it's recommended you learn them with a qualified TRE practitioner.

Quantitative electroencephalography (qEEG)

A qEEG is a diagnostic assessment which involves measuring brainwaves to see if they are behaving as expected. Research has shown they are effective at picking up post-concussion syndrome. The information can be presented as a brain map. Follow-up treatment often takes the form of neurofeedback.

Neurofeedback (NFB)

NFB, also called neurotherapy, is a type of biofeedback that presents real-time feedback from brain activity in order to reinforce healthy brain function. In other words, it is a technology that can improve brain function and mental well-being by providing the brain with direct, real-time feedback on how it is working. Typically, electrical activity from the brain is collected via sensors placed on the scalp using electro-encephalography (EEG), with feedback presented using video displays or sound.

Neurofeedback takes advantage of neuroplasticity and is based on the concept of operant conditioning (where new behaviour is learned through reward). Parts of the brain are re-trained to be more or less responsive via this reward principle. The brain is very flexible; if we do not use a circuit or we rely heavily on other circuits this can create an imbalance within the brain where, for example, the fear centres get activated more frequently at the expense of brain circuits that are responsible for rational higher-order thinking, problem solving and calmness. As such, neurofeedback trains the fear centres of the brain to be less responsive and draw upon other neural networks that may have become redundant.

Although the technology behind neurofeedback is complex and draws upon brain waves, the process is simple, painless and non-invasive. The process helps people to learn to alter their brain activity the same way we learn other skills, through feedback, practice and reward. In relation to brain injury, neurofeedback helps the individual exercise pathways to improve nervous system regulation and brain function.

In the early stages after a traumatic brain injury, neurofeedback can be helpful with the head pain that is often experienced, as well as with nausea, irritability, mental confusion and sleep difficulties. Over the longer term, neurofeedback can be helpful with energy levels, vigilance, effort fatigue, cognitive dysfunction traceable to the injury, sensory hypersensitivity and executive function. Over time, memory function may recover as well.

There is significant evidence supporting neurotherapy for the generalized treatment of mental disorders, and it has been practised for over four decades, although never gaining prominence in the medical mainstream. NFB has minimal side effects relatively, although some people have found that tapping into a state of calm can feel strange as it is a state that they are not familiar with. However, it is a long-term treatment plan, and the clinician works collaboratively with the client to optimize the neurofeedback settings. Margaret Ayers was one of the early neurofeedback practitioners to treat traumatic brain injury, and she achieved remarkable results with hundreds of patients, albeit with more severe injuries. Dr Jonathan Walker, a Dallas neurologist, observed significant improvement in 88 per cent of a group of 26 patients with mild closed-head traumatic brain injury. Every one of them who had held a job prior to their injury was able to resume productive employment after neurofeedback. The average number of neurofeedback sessions people undertook in as part of their treatment was 19.

There are a number of companies offering neurofeedback. As with many 'alternative' interventions, NHS funding is not available. I referred a number of my clients to Brain Train UK (www.braintainuk.com) and I have found that the neurofeedback complements the work we are doing in neuropsychology sessions.

Hyperbaric oxygen therapy (HBOT)

Hyperbaric oxygen therapy involves entering a pressurized chamber and breathing in pure oxygen for a set amount of time over a number of sessions. It has been claimed that this can help speed up healing of the brain and improve a number of the symptoms of injury, including headaches and cognitive impairments. Recent studies are varied in their findings about the efficacy of HBOT, however many individuals with brain injury report that it has helped them. You can find out more about HBOT and mild brain injury at <https://www.brainline. org/treatment-hub/hyperbaric-oxygen-therapy-hbot>

Low-level laser (light) therapy (LLLT) and red light therapy

Also known as photobiomodulation therapy, LLLT and red light therapy are showing promise as healing treatments for concussion. Light treatment may activate mitochondria and increase energy production as well as increasing blood flow, increasing neurogenesis, having neuroprotective benefits and reducing symptoms.

The Feldenkrais Method

The Feldenkrais Method is a type of exercise therapy devised by Moshe Feldenkrais during the mid 20th century. It is a method that teaches a variety of movement, self-awareness and mindfulness practices with an aim of reorganizing connections between the brain and body, which has a positive impact on body movement and psychological state. Having a greater awareness of the link between the mind and body can help a person to move in a way that is easier and more pleasurable.

Yoga therapy

Yoga therapy is more than going to a yoga class a few times a week. It is the application of yoga practices to assist with self-care for all, particularly those suffering with physical and mental health conditions. Yoga therapists are usually yoga teachers who have undertaken further comprehensive training and studies to become a yoga therapist. It has its own special training programme and yoga therapists usually work individually with clients using their knowledge of yoga practices and tools to assist their clients on a path to better health. For many, yoga has been associated with bringing a sense of calm through different breathing practices, body postures and movements as well as meditation. Yoga is seen to help people move out of sympathetic activation and into parasympathetic activation, which for people that are experiencing anxiety and trauma symptoms is highly beneficial. However, for those that present with low energy and have depressed mood, the target of their yoga therapy may be more about engaging in stimulating breathing and movement practices and getting them out of a chronic parasympathetic state into a more sympathetic activated state.

There is a wealth of scientific research supporting the use of yoga therapy for a range of physical and mental illnesses, and trauma experts champion its use for helping people suffering from PTSD. Given that many people with mTBI also have trauma symptoms and are in a state of sympathetic activation, yoga therapy can be a very powerful tool for helping people in their recovery journey. There is a yoga programme specially developed for people with brain injury created between Yoga International and the Love Your Brain Foundation (<www. loveyourbrain.com>).

Further information on yoga therapy and therapists from an established UK company can be found here: <www.themindedinstitute.com>

Ayurveda

Ayurveda is India's traditional medical system and complements yoga therapy. Along with traditional Chinese medicine (see below), it can be seen as the first integrated medicine and health system. According to Ayurveda each one of us has a unique constitution that shapes what we look like, how we think, how we respond to things in our environment and what types of illnesses and diseases we may be more vulnerable to experiencing. There are three constitution types (doshas) called Kapha, Pitta and Vata. Each has its own qualities that are borne out in a person when they are in balance and also when they are out of balance. For example, a person who is predominantly Pitta is typically focused, passionate and highly motivated (think type A personalities), but when out of balance will move more towards anger and aggressiveness, and is more likely to experience heart disease as a medical condition. People who are more Vata tend to be creative and have lots of energy, but can find it hard to focus on one thing. When out of balance these 'types' are more likely to develop diseases of the nervous system, including anxiety and insomnia. Ayurveda clinicians will 'prescribe' dietary and lifestyle habits that will help you keep in balance.

Often yoga therapists will have some knowledge of Ayurveda to help inform the best yoga practices and tools to help that individual move towards balance and away from disease and can really assist with creating an internal and external environment that supports physical, mental and spiritual wellness.

Chinese medicine

Chinese medicine is also an ancient medical system that has a wealth of knowledge and expertise in treating ill health in a more integrated way. While modern medicine tends to separate the brain from the body, use a reductionist view of human health and disease and focus on treatment rather than prevention, traditional medical systems prefer a holistic understanding view of health that reaches beyond the individual's body and mind and seeks to understand the world in which they live and how it impacts on their well-being. Acupuncture is just one of the many tools used in Chinese medicine to help treat imbalances and create optimized health.

Craniosacral therapy (CST)

Craniosacral therapy (CST) is a gentle hands-on treatment that may provide relief from a variety of symptoms and problems including headaches, neck pain and medication side effects as well as PCS.

The hands-on nature of the treatment helps to relieve stress responses in the central nervous system, assists in releasing tension in the connective tissue and muscles and promotes optimum blood flow. By supporting feelings of safety, gentle touch can reduce pain and boost health and immunity. Fascia is a body-wide connective network that covers all organs, glands, nerves, muscles, blood vessels, brain and spinal cord. CST is based on the idea that the body is interrelated at all levels. CST is thought to improve efficiency of biological processes through boosting inherent self-regulation and self-healing.

A CST session could be compared to massage therapy, except you stay fully clothed and the hands-on contact of the therapist is very light and non-manipulative. This light touch and fascial release may help your muscles and organs naturally relieve stress, which improves function. People often report feeling a sense of deep relaxation after a session which means their nervous system has been encouraged into a parasympathetic state.

Biodynamic craniosacral therapy (BCST) is an offshoot of CST that brings the relational field between the client and therapist more into focus while acknowledging the deepest foundations of the human system. Biodynamic craniosacral therapy takes a whole-person approach to healing and the interconnections of mind, body and spirit are deeply acknowledged. It is an effective form of treatment for a wide range of illnesses, helping to create the optimal conditions for health, encouraging vitality and facilitating a sense of well-being.

Below are the links to the UK and US practitioner directories:
<https://www.craniosacral.co.uk/practitioner-directory/>
<https://www.craniosacraltherapy.org/>
International Affiliation of Biodynamic Trainings (IABT)
<www.biodynamic-craniosacral.org>

Myofascial release therapy (MFR)

Myofascial release therapy is focused on treating and loosening the deep and surface fascia (the interconnective tissue) on the head and body. This can become dry and tight after a concussion, physical injury or trauma. Treatment can help to relieve stresses and strains to the fascia, leading to increased blood flow and pain reduction.

Art therapy

Art therapy enables a person to tap into their creative abilities and express themselves through an artistic medium. It can be helpful for allowing a person to explore and process emotions and feelings, contributing to mental well-being.

Music and sound therapy

Music and sound are known to have a calming and destressing effect. They can also evoke many different emotions and memories and can help with cognition and movement. You can either listen to or play music on your own or in a group. Alternatively, you could seek out a music and sound therapist to work with you one-to-one or in a group setting.

A specialism of music therapy is neurologic music therapy (NMT) which has been developed specifically to support people living with neurological conditions in terms of emotional, psychological, cognitive, communicative and social needs. It has been found to help with concentration and attentional skills as well as facilitating people to work with and tolerate strong emotions in the face of the challenges brought about by a neurological condition.

Psychology professionals

A qualified psychologist such as a clinical psychologist, counsellor or psychotherapist can help to support you with your emotional well-being and mental health. Some will have specialist knowledge of brain injury but even if they don't, their support can be very beneficial, especially if you are unable to access neuropsychology input.

Life coaching

Life coaching helps a person to manage change, consider and shape their future and move towards specific goals. Life coaching is not counselling or psychological support and is best undertaken at a later stage of recovery, when a person is in a position to take action in order to move their life forward.

PART TWO

PART TWO

8

Self-management techniques: focus on physical healing

This chapter, and the two following, are written solely by Anna based upon the treatment she has received, therapies she has partaken in and all the research that she has done since her injury to inform her recovery. While this and the next chapter have separated the focus into self-management techniques for physical and psychological symptoms, you will see that there is overlap in the tools and techniques provided. Many people find that managing physical symptoms has a positive impact on psychological symptoms and subsequently promotes healing of the mind, while working on healing the mind will have a positive impact on physical recovery.

Track your symptoms

Tracking allows you to pinpoint your main symptoms, identify possible triggers and plan your care and self-management. A symptom tracker can be used just for yourself, by a caregiver or you can share the information with your doctor and/or other medical professionals to help inform your treatment plan.

You can keep track of your symptoms either on a paper chart or spreadsheet like I did or you can use an online symptom tracker like the free one from Power of Patients, <www.power-ofpatients.com>. Founder Lynne Becker has over 25 years' experience in the medical sciences field, and direct experience after both her daughters suffered brain injuries. It takes a couple of minutes to set up and is intuitive and easy to use. You can track symptoms such as headaches, brain fog, dizziness, fatigue, blurred vision and so on, with the option to add your own. You can view the results online or print off a paper copy.

Sleep

Disrupted sleep patterns can lead to an exacerbation of concussion symptoms. Contributing factors to poor sleep include inflammation in the brain, hormonal issues, disruption of circadian rhythms, anxiety, pain and trauma. A person can find themselves in a vicious cycle of feeling exhausted during the day, having symptom flare-ups and lying awake at night, desperately trying to get to sleep.

The optimal amount of time for a good night's sleep is 7–8 hours. During sleep a number of important processes essential for good health take place in the brain, including the formation and organization of memories, processing of information, the clearing out of toxins and waste and cell repair. Research has shown that good quality sleep can improve a person's recovery outcomes after a concussion.

Not having enough sleep at night significantly affects how I function during the day, how bad my symptoms are, how much energy I have and how tired I feel. A build-up of poor sleep over time makes things even worse. Below I will share some of the things that have helped me to improve my sleep, which you might like to try:

1 Have a bedtime routine and aim to implement it every night so that it becomes a habit. Start to wind down at least an hour before you go to bed so that you feel rested at bedtime. Aim to be in bed by 10–10.30 p.m.

2 Don't eat too late – some nutrition experts say within three hours of going to bed. This gives you time to digest your food before you go to sleep.

3   If possible, don't nap for too long in the day. Short cat naps of around 15 minutes or so can be as effective as longer sleeps. There may be times during the day you feel you need to rest for longer and that's fine but try not to do it too often as it can make it harder to fall asleep at night.

4   Do exercise and keep active in the day if you can but don't do vigorous exercise too close to bedtime. Gentle exercise such as stretching is OK and can help you wind down.

5   Stop using a screen – computer, TV, mobile phone or similar devices – at least an hour before bedtime. If you do use a screen in the evening, then use a light filter which blocks the blue light. Blue light restricts the production of melatonin, the hormone that helps you fall asleep. There are various apps to block blue light, including F.lux (<www.justgetflux.com>).

6   Don't watch or read the news before bedtime. Humans have a negativity bias which means we're hardwired to focus more on negative experiences rather than positive or neutral ones. A lot of the news is about challenging events and can trigger negative thoughts and feelings. There are just as many, if not more, good things going on in the world that never get reported on.

7   Some herbal teas are known to help with sleep, such as chamomile, lavender, lemon balm and passionflower. There are also sleep blends available. Check for contraindications before taking, especially if you're on medication or are pregnant.

8   Don't drink alcohol or coffee or tea for several hours before bedtime (some say from midday onwards) as caffeine stays in your system for hours and can keep you awake at night.

9   Write out a to-do list and plan in the evening for the following day.

10 Lay out your clothes for the following day.

11   Take a shower or have a relaxing bath at bedtime, maybe with some essential oils, bubble bath or Epsom salts.

12   Ensure your curtains or blinds completely block out the light or use blackout blinds so that your room is really dark.

13   Make sure your room is at a comfortable temperature. Open the window a little so the air circulates and stays fresh. In summer, use a fan if it's very hot.

14   Change your bedding regularly so that it's clean and comfortable.

15   Keep your room clutter free and keep it as a haven.

16   Listen to a meditation, audio CD, binaural beats or gentle music.

17   Read a book, especially fiction.

18   If you have a spiritual practice, do that.

19   Before you fall asleep, think of a few things from the day you're grateful for.

20   If your mind's active, keep a notepad and pen by your bed so you can write down anything you don't want to forget.

21   Use earplugs to block out any noise.

22   Wear a sleep mask to block out any light.

23   If you can't get to sleep after about 20 minutes or so, or you wake in the night and can't get back to sleep, read or get up and do something. Or try doing a body scan or meditating.

24   Use a sleep spray on your pillow such as lavender or a special blend of essential oils; I use Tisserand Sleep Spray (<www.tisserand.com>).

Follow a morning routine

You might also want to create a morning routine. Routines add certainty, predictability and a degree of control into your day and relieve some of the energy requirements of your brain. My morning routine, which I do before breakfast and getting ready, varies. Experiment and try out different things and see what works for you. Here are some suggestions:

1   Drink a large glass of water so you're hydrated.
2   Have a smoothie or a hot drink such as a cup of herbal tea.
3   If you feel hungry, eat a healthy snack such as fruit.
4   Check your to-do list and plan for the day.
5   Read part of an interesting or inspiring book or watch or listen to something enjoyable or inspiring.
6   Meditate, reflect, pray or practise mindfulness.
7   Do some breathing exercises.
8   Journal.
9   Listen to relaxing music.
10 Think of at least five things you're grateful for.
11 Do some exercise or stretching.
12 Go outside, either in the garden or for a walk, so you move and get some fresh air and vitamin D.

Diet and nutrition

Good nutrition is crucial for a healthy brain. An adult brain weighs approximately 3 lb or 1.3–1.4 kg and represents only approximately 2 per cent of a person's bodyweight. However, it uses up more energy than any other organ in the body at around 20 per cent of a person's total daily energy reserves. The brain is made up of approximately 75 per cent water and approximately 60 per cent fat. So, it's vital that we look after it, feed it the right nutrients and keep it hydrated in order for it to function optimally, especially if it's been injured.

The brain is connected to the digestive system by the vagus nerve. This is known as 'the gut–brain axis'. It refers to the bi-directional communication link between the brain and the digestive system, which has its own nervous system called the 'enteric nervous system' and contains 500 million neurons as well as neurotransmitters. For this reason, the gut is sometimes referred to as 'the second brain'. For an explanation of and further insight into this subject, see Chapter 9,'The Gut–Brain Axis', in the book, *Why Isn't My Brain Working?* by Dr Datis Kharrazian.

Eating a brain-healthy diet will, among other things, help to:

- reduce inflammation in the brain and body
- repair the gut lining which may have become permeable – 'leaky' – after your injury
- reduce toxic substances crossing the blood–brain barrier
- regulate blood sugar levels
- reduce oxidative stress
- improve functioning of the mitochondria, which improves overall energy
- provide essential nutrients for health and healing
- improve the quality of the gut flora.

I recommend the book '*How to Feed a Brain*' by brain injury survivor Cavin Balaster. His nutritional guidelines include some elements of both paleolithic and ketogenic diets. He refers to '*The Wahls Protocol*', a paleolithic dietary protocol developed by Dr Terry Wahls, who has managed to reverse her multiple sclerosis symptoms. Both their approaches focus primarily on maximizing nutritional value, optimizing the function of the mitochondria – the energy producers of the brain and body's cells – and regenerating myelin, which insulates neurons in the brain.

Cavin Balaster suggests making the dietary changes in his book for 60 days and then continuing to stick with the general principles while re-introducing certain foods and seeing how that goes. The diet contains meat but if you're vegetarian then you could try following a plant-based brain-healthy diet such as the MIND diet or '*The 30-Day Alzheimer's Solution*' by Drs Dean and Ayesha Sherzai. You'll need to take any special dietary require-ments you have into consideration. You may decide to work with a dietician; some dieticians work with people with brain injuries.

I followed quite a strict diet for a couple of months and then I relaxed things, little by little. Today, I still mainly base what I eat on the principles of the Paleolithic, Mediterranean and Ketogenic diets. In my personal experience, changing my diet was a big game-changer for my recovery.

Below are some suggestions for a brain-healthy diet after a concussion, based on 'How to Feed a Brain', other sources (some of which are mentioned in the 'Resources' section at the end of this book) and my own experience. I am not a dietician, so please do your own research into diet, especially as everyone has different preferences and you may have certain dietary requirements. If appropriate, please consult your healthcare provider and/or a dietician.

1 It's recommended that adults drink approximately eight glasses of water per day. Swap fruit juices and sweet drinks for water and only have the occasional glass of real fruit juice. A cup of coffee or tea is OK and mushroom coffee is a healthy alternative. Certain teas have health benefits, for example chai, camomile, green tea, peppermint and tulsi. Check if you have any health issues that make it inadvisable for you to drink herbal teas.

2 It's best not to drink alcohol in the early part of your recovery. Everyone's tolerance level to alcohol after an mTBI is different, so if you do start to drink again, then build up slowly. Personally, over five years post-injury, I still only have the odd glass of wine very rarely as I find I'm still sensitive to alcohol and invariably feel quite hungover the next day. You will find what works best for you.

3 Eat a variety of fresh fruit and vegetables every day. They contain antioxidants, minerals, phytochemicals and vitamins. Fruits with a low Glycemic Index (GI) cause a lower, slower rise in blood sugar. These include apples, bananas, blueberries, cherries, grapefruit, pears, oranges, raspberries and strawberries. Eat leafy green vegetables such as kale, romaine lettuce, spinach and watercress; colourful vegetables

such as beetroot and radishes; cruciferous vegetables such as broccoli and cauliflower; and sulphur-rich produce such as garlic, onions and cooked mushrooms. Raw fruit and vegetables are delicious in smoothies.

4 Cut out or reduce your intake of processed foods, such as fast foods, which can be inflammatory and are low in nutritional value.

5 Eliminate or decrease your intake of added sugar to keep it to a minimum. Glucose is the main form of energy for your body's cells, organs, tissues and the neurons in your brain, but too much added sugar is bad for you. The American Heart Association states that naturally occurring sugars in foods are enough and no extra sugar is necessary. The maximum amount of added sugar recommended by the NHS is seven teaspoons per day for an adult. I suggest keeping below that. There's more sugar than you realize in foods such as cereals, sauces and some 'low-fat' and 'healthy' snacks.

6 Limit your salt intake; the WHO recommends just under a teaspoon per day.

7 Good fats are anti-inflammatory and are essential for the brain to function well. Exchange industrial-made trans fats for healthy fats. Avocado oil, coconut oil, virgin olive oil or ghee are good for cooking. A tablespoon or so of butter is OK, especially if it's grass-fed, but avoid margarine. Avocadoes are a good source of healthy fat. Avoid so-called 'low-fat' foods as they often contain sugar or sweeteners.

8 Oily fish such as mackerel, salmon, sardines, trout and tuna contain protein for healthy function of neurotransmitters as well as omega-3 fatty acids which are essential for building a healthy brain and help with both learning and memory. Aim for 2–3 portions a week.

9 Seeds, including chia, flax, pumpkin and sunflower, contain protein, omega-3s, fibre, minerals, vitamins and antioxidants. Have them on their own or on cereals or salads.

10   Good quality meat, such as beef, chicken, lamb and turkey, contains folate, vitamins and protein which help create enzymes, hormones and other chemicals in our bodies. It's also essential for the healing and repair of our cells. Meat can be inflammatory, though, especially processed meats such as bacon, ham and salami, so it's best to avoid those.

11   Bone broth, used as stock or soup, contains many nutrients and may be good for the digestive system, and helps to calm inflammation. If you're vegetarian or vegan, try vegetable broth instead.

12   Consider reducing dairy because it can be inflammatory. Also, some people are intolerant to casein, which can result in allergic reactions such as swelling or itching, and/or lactose, which can cause digestive issues, bloating and stomach pain. I cut out dairy completely for a few weeks and then gradually re-introduced it, though I eat less than I used to as a matter of personal preference and I generally now drink lactose-free milk. You can substitute dairy with oat, coconut, almond or one of the many plant-based milks and foods such as vegan cheese and coconut yoghurt. Cottage cheese, feta cheese, mozzarella and Greek yoghurt are better options if you do consume dairy. If you're concerned about having a low calcium intake due to reducing dairy, then be assured that calcium is contained in various foods, including leafy green vegetables, such as spinach, kale and bok choy; broccoli; cabbage; watercress; oranges and orange juice; some cereals; oatmeal; nuts; sesame seeds; beans such as baked beans; and white beans; chick peas; and tofu.

13   Eggs contain choline, an essential nutrient needed for synthesis of the neurotransmitter acetylcholine that helps regulate memory and mood. They're a good source of B6, B12 and folate. They contain cholesterol but some cholesterol is necessary in our diets for building cells, making hormones and creating myelin membrane growth.

14   Carbohydrates provide energy for the body, but reduce portion size and avoid refined carbohydrates such as white bread, white rice, white pasta and baked goods.

15   Remove or limit gluten as it can cause food sensitivities, inflammation and contribute to symptoms such as brain fog and fatigue. Gluten is found in foods containing wheat, such as bread, cakes and biscuits, cereal, some grains and pasta. Eat gluten-free versions of these foods or try alternatives.

16   Legumes such as beans, peas and lentils contain protein, B vitamins, minerals and fibre. Rinse them thoroughly and soak for a few hours or overnight if possible before cooking as they contain lectins which can cause inflammation of the gut lining.

17   Incorporate herbs and spices into your cooking. Good ones include turmeric, paprika, ginger, parsley, coriander, basil, thyme, oregano and cinnamon.

18   Keep a supply of healthy snacks such as apples, blueberries, grapes, seaweed, avocados, hummus, carrot sticks, celery sticks, small squares of 70 per cent dark chocolate and protein bars.

19   If you're going out somewhere, take healthy snacks and water with you so you can eat or drink if you start feeling tired or hungry.

20   Consider using a slow cooker at home so you can make simple, nutritious meals very easily.

Supplements

If you are on other medication, always consult your prescribing physician before taking supplements.

About four months post-concussion, when I started to make changes to my diet, I decided to try some natural supplements. I took various ones at different stages of my recovery and generally found them to be very effective in alleviating and helping me to manage my symptoms. Today, I try to meet my nutritional needs through food and drink as much as possible so I take relatively few of them.

To learn more about supplements for optimal brain health, look at some of the books and resources, especially under 'Concussion Recovery Books' and 'Nutrition and Supplements' in the Resources and Further Reading section at the end of this book.

Do speak to your doctor or healthcare provider before taking any supplements and do your own research too, to check for any possible side effects and allergic reactions, recommended safe dosage, potential negative interactions of supplements and medication and contraindications, such as pregnancy.

Below, I'll briefly share a quick overview of the main supplements which helped me.

Alpha-lipoic acid

Alpha-lipoic acid is a fatty acid involved in energy metabolism and has powerful anti-oxidative and anti-inflammatory properties.

Ashwagandha

Ashwagandha is an adaptogenic herb, in other words, it helps your body to adapt better to stress. I found it helped me to feel calmer and more resilient and to sleep better, though it occasionally made me feel a little drowsy at times during the day.

Bulletproof Brain Octane C8 MCT Oil

I take a tablespoon of Brain Octane Oil most days, either on its own or in coffee or on salads. It makes me feel more alert and focused and gives me an energy boost. It's a medium-chain triglyceride (MCT) oil, so it can help to increase the production of ketones – an alternative energy source to glucose – for your brain, and it's absorbed quickly into the bloodstream. Start with a teaspoon and build up gradually to having more.

Boswellia

Boswellia, also known as Indian frankincense, has anti-inflammatory properties. I've used it successfully to reduce chronic pain.

CBD oil

I found CBD oil beneficial for pain relief, anxiety relief and better clarity and focus. Much scientific research is currently going on regarding CBD oil as an effective treatment for concussion due to its potential antioxidant, anti-inflammatory and neuroprotective qualities. It's not psychoactive and is generally believed to be safe. It's legal in the UK (as long as it contains no THC, the psychoactive component), Canada and most states in the US but rules vary in different countries around the world, so do make sure to check. I've used the brands Cannabigold and Charlotte's Web.

Cognizin Citicoline

Citicoline is a nutrient found in the body that's essential for good brain function. Cognizin Citicoline is the brand name of a supplement that has been shown in studies to improve attention, focus, memory and energy production in the brain.

CoQ10

Coenzyme Q10 (CoQ10) is a naturally occurring nutrient and antioxidant in the body that can be supplemented. It may increase blood supply to the brain, increase energy production and reduce neurodegeneration.

Curcumin

Curcumin is a compound with powerful anti-inflammatory properties and I've found it very effective at reducing chronic pain. It also increases blood flow in the brain and may improve focus and memory and have neuroprotective properties. It's a more bioavailable form of the bright-yellow spice, turmeric, which means it's better absorbed into the bloodstream. Certain brands of the supplement form of curcumin claim to have increased bioavailability, or you can take it with black pepper to increase its efficacy.

Feverfew

Feverfew is a medicinal plant, believed to be a natural painkiller and anti-inflammatory, that can be bought in pill form. I've used it successfully to treat my migraine headaches.

L-carnitine

L-carnitine is a naturally occurring nutrient in the body that can also be taken in supplement form. Acetyl-L-carnitine (ALCAR) is supposedly the best form to take for your brain. It may increase the function and energy production of the mitochondria and may also contribute to healthy brain function.

L-glutamine

L-glutamine is an amino acid that can be taken as a dietary supplement, usually in powdered form, that may support gut health and healing.

L-theanine

L-theanine is an amino acid that occurs in tea and can be taken as a supplement. I've found it helpful for reducing anxiety and for making me feel generally calmer.

Magnesium

Magnesium is a mineral with a whole host of health benefits, including contributing to the healthy functioning of the nervous system, regulating mood and reducing anxiety, fatigue and muscle stiffness. I've taken it in the form magnesium citrate, which is supposedly more easily absorbed into the bloodstream.

Omega-3 fish oil

Dr Michael Lewis of the Brain Health Education and Research Institute in the US has developed a high-dose fish oil protocol for concussion and brain injury recovery. Good quality fish oil contains omega-3 fatty acids containing EPA and a higher level of DHA. EPA helps to regulate cellular inflammation while DHA helps to maintain nerve cell structure and function. For more information, go to the website <www.brainhealtheducation.org>. I noticed a marked improvement in brain function after following the protocol.

Rhodiola rosea

Rhodiola rosea is an adaptogenic herb, claimed to help the body regulate stress. I found it very effective for making me feel more alert and focused and for lifting the brain fog that I frequently experienced.

Vitamins and minerals

For some time I took a daily multivitamin and mineral supplement in order to ensure that I was getting good levels of essential vitamins and minerals into my body for optimal mental and physical health. The main ones were the B vitamins, vitamin C, vitamin D3 and vitamin E. In addition, I was recommended to take 400 mg per day of vitamin B2 (riboflavin) for the vestibular migraines I was experiencing. The vitamin B2 supplements really helped to reduce the number and severity of migraines and vertigo I was having.

Exercise

The current general medical advice for people immediately in the days following a concussion is to rest, both physically and cognitively, to allow the brain and body time to heal, and not to return straight away to sports and exercise.

If you play competitive sports, team sports or take part in sport at a high level, then it's essential to get cleared for return to play by your coach and a doctor. The Mayo Clinic website states that a person should never return to play or energetic activity if they still have signs or symptoms of a concussion. Another concussion sustained shortly after the first one can lead to second-impact syndrome, which can be fatal.

After an initial rest and healing period of about 24 to 48 hours in the acute phase, many concussion experts now believe it's beneficial to start gradually building up tolerance to activities.

Some concussion health professionals recommend starting some form of graded exercise less than a week after injury, depending on symptom severity. The 'Buffalo Concussion Treadmill Test' (BCTT) is a concussion protocol developed by John J. Leddy and Professor Barry Willer at the University of Buffalo, USA, which helps people increase their exercise tolerance with graded exercise according to their symptom threshold by monitoring the heart rate threshold (HRT). Usually performed by two health professionals, the test shows the amount of aerobic exercise it's safe for a person to do after their concussion. The person would then follow a graded exercise plan, exercising regularly and consistently at just below their threshold of symptoms, monitoring their progress and building up gradually. It's best to have guidance from a health professional on this, especially in the early days of recovery. Google the BCTT or go to <www.ubortho.com/services/concussion-management-center/> for more information.

Some of the benefits of exercise, when carried out in an appropriate way for a person's age, general fitness, circumstances and stage of recovery after a concussion, include:

- an increase in blood flow to the brain
- the heart working harder to deliver oxygen and nutrients in the bloodstream to the muscles and different parts of the body

- an increase in the number of mitochondria in the brain and body, resulting in more energy
- increased muscle strength
- a more regulated and resilient nervous system
- improved proprioception – the body's sense of its position in space
- better balance
- improved posture
- less stiffness
- an increase in BDNF (brain-derived neurotrophic factor), a protein that promotes neurogenesis (the growth of new brain cells) and communication between neurons
- an increase in endorphins leading to less pain and an overall improvement in mood and sense of well-being
- better cognitive function, including faster processing skills, improved memory and less brain fog
- fewer symptoms
- a faster recovery time.

As the result of a concussion, some people suffer from a condition called dysautonomia, which is dysfunction of the autonomic nervous system. Symptoms include dizziness, exercise intolerance, fast heart rate and high blood pressure. It can be diagnosed by checking heart rate variability (HRV), which is best done by a specialist. You can find out more on the website: <www.dysautonomiainternational.org>

PoTS (Postural Tachycardia Syndrome) is a form of dysautonomia experienced by some concussion survivors. Symptoms occur when a person is standing up and are generally only relieved by lying down. These include chest pain, light-headedness, shaking and temperature sensitivity. Check out the website, <www.potsuk.org>, for advice on self-management techniques and exercise. If you've been diagnosed with dysautonomia or PoTS then it's best to take a more conservative approach to exercise and work with a specialist.

Exercise has played an important role in my own recovery and I always feel so much more alive after I've done some. Initially, as I was in a lot of pain, my physiotherapist gave me gentle exercises to move my neck, arms and torso and to help me walk properly again. I practised the exercises at home every day in between appointments but apart from that I thought that resting would be the best thing to do as I was afraid that exercise would make me worse. On reflection, I wish I'd exercised sooner as my posture deteriorated, my proprioception (ability of my body to sense movement and its location in space) was poor, I became very stiff and my pain persisted.

After some time, encouraged and inspired by some people in a Facebook post-concussion support group I was in, I decided to start walking up and down my garden every day and then I progressed to jogging, then running short distances. I went for short walks in the countryside near my house, joined a local stretch class and followed a Pilates DVD my physiotherapist recommended. At that stage, I didn't understand about exercising at a sub-optimal level so I'd often get symptomatic and then not feel able to exercise again for at least a couple of days.

After about a year, on Dr Pradhan's recommendation, I started a gentle online exercise program, 'Movingness' (<www.movingness.com>), created by Peter Appel, an embodiment and movement teacher. I started with very small movements, building up gently to more strenuous ones, using a combination of specific movements, dance, mindfulness and stretching. The aim of these exercises was to calm down the nervous system at times and stimulate it at others. I began to be able to move in ways I'd been unable to for so long. For the first time, exercise didn't cause symptom flare-ups and I was able to gradually build up my exercise tolerance.

Many people find yoga helpful after a brain injury because it combines movement and stretching with breathwork and mindfulness. I've recently taken up qigong, a gentle Chinese practice based on similar principles, that helps me to feel calmer and more energized. I alternate this with doing more aerobic forms of exercise when I can, usually weights, resistance training, high intensity interval training (HIIT), swimming or vigorous walking.

Two years post-injury, I resumed my favourite sport, swimming, and over time I've worked up to swimming up to 40 lengths at a time and I've also been river swimming, bodysurfing in the sea and canoeing. For me, the benefits of being in the water include relaxation, pain relief, improved coordination and mobility and better focus.

I was also able to ride a bike again, which made me so happy. Since then, I've had a go at a few new activities, such as wall climbing, high ropes and even a zipwire. I wanted to do as much as I could to challenge myself, heal my vestibular system and improve my general fitness levels.

Four years post-injury, I was able to climb steep hills on holiday in the Peak District and around the same time, I took part in a fundraising walk for Headway, the UK brain injury charity, covering 26.2 km over three weeks and walking ten miles on one day.

It took me a relatively long time to regain my fitness levels, partly due to my injuries, my life circumstances and lack of knowledge of what to do. Everyone's journey to fitness after a concussion will vary and no two timeframes will be the same. There's no one-size-fits-all recovery training programme and there are no guarantees but the important thing to remember is that exercise is possible and beneficial, both physically and mentally, after a concussion. Many people go on to achieve a good level of fitness, with some attaining their pre-injury fitness levels and others going well beyond.

Here are some suggestions for exercising, once you're able to:

1 Keep moving. Build regular short breaks – and if possible longer ones – into your day. If you're able to, do get up and

move about regularly – at least for about a few minutes every 45 minutes or so. Or do some simple neck, shoulder, back and arm exercises if you need to stretch. Start with exercises sitting in a chair or lying down if that's all you're able to do.

2 Simple day-to-day activities all add up and help increase your energy levels, for example going up the stairs a bit more quickly, making yourself fetch things from another room, watering the flowers in the garden or walking a little further than you usually would.

3 It's better to do a small amount of exercise every day – even just 5–10 minutes – than a long workout once a week. Do whatever you can. Build up gradually and at your own pace. Start with a walk outside or something fairly gentle and build up. Aim to exercise at a suboptimal level, where your symptoms aren't exacerbated. If you can work up to 30 minutes, three or four times a week, that's great. You may wish to do more.

4 Some people find weights and resistance training helpful for alleviating post-concussion symptoms.

5 HIIT or mid intensity interval training (MIIT) alternates short bursts of aerobic energy with short periods of going at a slower pace. An example of HIIT would be to do a minute or a minute and a half of strenuous, high-impact exercise such as running on the spot or running, then a minute of walking and so on, for about 10–15 minutes.

6 Crossing the midline exercises are good for improving bilateral coordination, balance and spatial and visual issues.

7 Buy some home equipment such as a balance board, weights or resistance bands.

8 Consider using a tracker such as a Fitbit or a heart rate variability tracker to monitor your fitness and progress.

9 Do forms of exercise you enjoy, rather than doing something you think you ought to do or that everyone else is doing. To motivate you, you could join a local class or gym, watch an exercise DVD or YouTube videos or join an online program.

10 If you're struggling with more energetic forms of exercise, then switch to or alternate with gentler forms such as yoga, Pilates, qigong, tai chi or stretching.

Develop self-awareness around how you feel when you exercise so that you get better at judging when to push yourself a little more to the next stage or when to pull back if you've overdone things. Ideally, you want to be exercising at a point where you don't trigger symptoms. However, if you do experience increased symptoms, then concussion specialist Dr Cameron Marshall says it's not a sign of further damage to the brain; the injury happened in the past and you're not reinjuring yourself. While a flare-up of symptoms can be very unpleasant, it's temporary and will pass and isn't to be feared. Fear will make things worse and hold you back. He explains that if you don't challenge yourself physically, then you'll stay at the level you're at and won't make progress. It's a fine balance to achieve and you won't always get it right, but over time you'll generally get better at figuring out how much physical exertion you can comfortably do. Pace yourself; it takes time to increase your activity and fitness levels. If you have any concerns or questions regarding exercise after a concussion, speak to your healthcare provider.

Dealing with noise and light sensitivity

Two common problems for people who have had a concussion are light and noise sensitivity. These disorientating experiences can cause dizziness, headaches and other symptoms. Triggers can include bright sun, screens, busy roads, busy open spaces and noisy indoor places such as shopping malls, restaurants or sports facilities. Examples of triggers at home could be the TV, computer, people talking loudly or the sound of pans banging in the kitchen.

If you experience either light or sound sensitivity, do tell your doctor or healthcare provider. It may be that you have a vision, ear, balance or vestibular issue which can be treated.

You may, also, like me, suffer from vestibular migraines (find out more at <www.vestibularmigraine.co.uk>). The treatment for BPPV and balance that I had with a neuro-physiotherapist partly helped me to overcome noise and light sensitivity. I can't say exactly when things improved further for me, it was just a gradual process. Even today, I do occasionally experience one or the other but it doesn't usually last long.

Notice if there are particular environments or situations in which you experience noise or light sensitivity. Notice if you experience anxiety beforehand, in anticipation of being in one of these environments. Bring awareness to factors such as whether you're tired, didn't sleep well the night before or are feeling especially stressed or upset about something. Tracking your symptoms can really help.

Here are some simple things you can try to reduce your sensitivity to light and sound:

- Wear sunglasses or glasses with coloured lenses if it's bright (available from <www.happyeye.co.uk>).
- Wear earplugs (like the 'Isolate' or 'Calmer' ones from <www.flareaudio.com>) or noise-cancelling headphones.
- If you're out and about, talk to yourself internally about the situation and tell yourself you don't need to worry, you can handle this, you will be OK. If necessary, you can usually find somewhere to pause and sit down.
- Do some deep breathing for at least 30 seconds to a minute.
- If you're with people, let them know you're struggling so they have a better understanding of what you're experiencing and so you and they can make adjustments.
- Keep implementing the pillars of a healthy lifestyle such as getting a good night's sleep, mindfulness, meditation, exercise, healthy eating and positive social contact. This will help to create a more balanced nervous system that won't get so easily overloaded and overstimulated, and if it does, it will return to a state of equilibrium more quickly.

Concussion expert Dr Cameron Marshall recommends gradually building up exposure to bright, noisy environments to allow your brain to become accustomed to them. I did this and it worked, especially after getting my vision and balance issues seen to, and also as my physical pain decreased. It's best not to force it or go for too long as the repercussions can set you back for a while. If you do have a setback, don't let it put you off completely; keep experimenting. Try again when you feel ready, but maybe in a less triggering environment and for less time, and perhaps ask a supportive person to go with you.

Some people have tinnitus and hyperacusis after a concussion, and for these conditions it's advisable to seek specialist help, for example from an ear, nose and throat specialist. Additionally, some of the lifestyle practices mentioned in this book may help with managing these conditions.

Screens, social media and technology

The internet, social media and technology can be great for staying in contact with friends, researching recovery information and connecting with others dealing with concussion symptoms in online groups. However, there can be some challenges using technology after a concussion, including triggering symptoms, difficulty of use and communication misunderstandings. Below are a few tips for being online:

- Limit the length of time you spend online and choose times of day when you feel most alert.
- Build up slowly when using screens. Know your limits and recognize when you're starting to struggle. Even if you can only manage five minutes at a time, have a go, stop and try again later or another day.
- Using a blue light filter on your device minimizes disruption to your circadian rhythm and prevents screen glare, especially

early in the morning and in the evenings. I recommend downloading f.lux (<www.justgetflux.com>). Alternatively, wear glasses with coloured lenses (from <www.happyeye.co.uk>). Or you can use a screen overlay (available from <www.thedyslexiashop.co.uk>). If you're having trouble reading text on a page, you can put a coloured overlay over the text, available from The Dyslexia Shop or an ophthalmologist.

- Your head weighs approximately 5 kg or 11 lbs and it pulls forwards when you look at a screen. Take regular breaks from screens and get up and wander about and stretch a bit. Move your head from side to side from time to time and pull it back to avoid putting strain on your neck. Notice your posture and make sure you're sitting up straight.

- If you consistently find it hard to use screens, then you may have a problem with your eyes, neck or vestibular system so do make an appointment with a specialist to have this checked out.

- Notice how you feel when you're using social media. Ask yourself the question: 'Am I feeling better or worse about myself as a result of seeing this?' Comparing yourself to others – either healthy people or those sharing progress of their recoveries – may make you feel down. If you regularly feel worse after being on social media then take a break from it for a while.

- Joining an online concussion support group can be a very positive experience, providing you with good advice and helping you to feel less alone. Some of the down sides are that some people can be negative, share upsetting information, say insensitive things or give advice that may not be right for you. So be discerning. You can always pull back from a group for a while or leave if you find things get too much.

- You choose who you follow and who you're friends with on social media. While genuine and long-lasting relationships can be made, you can always unfollow, remove or block someone if you feel uncomfortable.

Therapeutic aids and equipment for use at home

There are many different aids you can use at home to help you with your recovery, available on Amazon or elsewhere online. Below are the ones I've personally used and found helpful:

- A massage ball, tennis ball or foam roller can be used for trigger point therapy or myofascial release therapy. This is very effective for relieving tension, muscle spasms and trigger points (painful knots) that form in the muscles, particularly in the head, neck, shoulders and back. Place the ball or roller either behind you on a wall or under you if you're lying on the floor, for roughly 30 to 60 seconds at a time, and lean the area of discomfort against it. Repeat if required. There's also an excellent self-massage and trigger point device called a Body Back Buddy. Alternatively, you can just press your fingers on tense areas that you can reach, such as your temples or neck, for 10 seconds to a minute at a time (or gently rub the area). Don't press too hard but apply pressure and then gently release it to a point where you're still applying pressure but not too much. There are free articles online and YouTube videos showing you how to do this.

Other home aids I've used and recommend (depending on your symptoms) are:

- acupressure mat and pillow
- balance board
- cervical neck stretcher
- cold pack (a small one to strap around your forehead or neck; a larger one to lie on; keep in the freezer)
- cold and heat spray, such as Deep Heat and Deep Freeze, which you can alternate on painful areas
- ibuprofen gel
- Dizzyclear pillow and accompanying book (for treatment of dizziness and vertigo)

- neck hammock
- posture corrector
- spiky massage ball to stimulate blood flow
- heated wheat pack for head, neck and shoulder pain
- yoga mat for exercise
- the 'C-Rod' (available from <u>concussionrecovery.net</u>) for home use to diagnose concussion and treat a number of associated vision problems. (It's been recommended to me but I've not used it.)

9

Self-management techniques: focus on healing the mind and body

Relationship with your mind and body

About two years after my accident, my GP recommended I take a mind–body approach to the chronic pain and some of the lingering post-concussion symptoms I was experiencing and referred me to an osteopath. After working with the osteopath for a couple of months, I subsequently worked with two mind–body coaches. Dr Pradhan also took a mind–body approach in her work with me, which was especially helpful as she also had specialist knowledge of concussion. I've read lots of books, listened to podcasts and watched videos on the subject as well.

Taking a mind–body approach to healing means acknowledging that the body and mind are not two separate entities but are interconnected, affecting each other and functioning together. What's going on in your head – in your brain and mind – will affect your body, and vice versa. Restoring the health of both is essential.

Understanding the link between the mind and body has been one of the positive things that has come out of my injury and I'm grateful for the knowledge that I now have. Applying this over the last few years has significantly contributed to my healing, including improved physical fitness, a reduction in anxiety and chronic pain, and a stronger mindset. Taking this approach will give you a sense of having greater control over your situation and make you feel more empowered.

The mind–body connection and chronic pain

Persistent pain is a common symptom of post-concussion syndrome. When it comes to the mind–body connection in relation to pain, the key thing to note is that all pain is interpreted, processed and created initially in the brain. The brain itself can't feel pain but it sends messages to different parts of the body to activate pain. Initially pain is caused to alert the body to take care of an injured area and to encourage it to heal. Usually, healing will happen in a matter of a few weeks or months. In the case of chronic pain, however, the brain can continue to signal pain to an area even though the threat has passed and the injury has healed. This type of pain, where neural pathways in the brain have been activated, is sometimes referred to as neuroplastic pain.

After my concussion, I developed pain sensitization. This means that the nerves carrying pain signals from the site of my original injury to my brain and the areas of painful sensation in my brain had become activated for a long time, creating a vicious cycle of pain. I had migraines or headaches every day for many months and for over five years I've had pain down the right-hand side of my body.

I've noticed that the pain often gets worse during times of emotional stress or if I've pushed myself too hard. There's a growing scientific understanding of the link between emotions and pain.

I've had some pain-free days, and there are a number of things that help to reduce or eliminate the pain, such as taking certain supplements, doing exercise, journaling, pacing myself, getting a good night's sleep and so on.

Below are some mind–body exercises you can do to help with chronic pain:

1 Sitting or lying down in a quiet room, do a gentle body scan. Then, focus on a part of your body which is in pain. Notice what comes to mind when you focus on this area. What

thoughts are you having? What emotions do you feel? Could something have triggered an increase in the level of pain? You may find it helpful afterwards to journal about your experience. This gets it out of your system and helps you to understand and process things.

2 Following on from 1, switch to focusing on an area of your body where you don't feel pain. Notice the contrast. After a while switch between the two different areas. See if you can bring some of the thoughts and feelings associated with the area not in pain to the painful area. Do this a few times. Either just make a mental note of your observations or you can write it down later.

3 Imagine a time when you didn't have any pain. How did you feel? What could you do? What did your life look like? Imagine yourself feeling like that now. Repeating this exercise regularly will activate different pathways in your brain.

If you're struggling with chronic pain, I recommend using the 'Curable' app (<www.curablehealth.com>) which combines techniques such as journaling, meditation, mindfulness and education as a way of understanding, reducing and in some cases eliminating pain. I also recommend reading the book '*Unlearn Your Pain*' by Dr Howard Schubiner to understand chronic pain better and learn practical ways to reduce it. Dr Schubiner clearly explains the fundamentals of neuroplastic pain and how neural pathways of pain can sometimes become established in the brains of some people who experience chronic pain. He shares a number of techniques and strategies to reduce and eliminate pain. I believe having a concussion adds another dimension to his explanations and approach but I think in general his advice and insights are still very helpful if your pain resulted from your head injury. In addition, Sheldon Press publishes the book *Chronic Pain: The Drug-free Way* by Phil Sizer, which also takes a holistic approach to addressing chronic pain.

Driving

Don't drive if you've had a concussion or if you continue to experience symptoms longer term. Do discuss driving with your doctor. In the UK you need to notify the DVLA if you've had a brain injury. If you live outside the UK then you'll need to find out what the requirements are with regards to notifying the appropriate driving and vehicle licensing agency in your country.

Cognitive rest versus cognitive strategies

The current medical advice is to rest for at least 24–48 hours post-injury and limit cognitive activities such as using a computer screen, reading, watching television or playing computer games in order to give the brain time to heal after being injured. The Mayo Clinic website refers to 'relative rest' and does not recommend complete rest, in other words, lying down in a dark room and doing absolutely nothing for days on end. Although this largely used to be the advice given to concussion patients, while it's important to rest the brain, prolonged complete rest is now not considered to be the best course of action for recovery.

As with physical exercise, it's now recommended by medical professionals that after 48 hours or so, a person gradually builds up their levels of activity at a pace that doesn't exacerbate symptoms. Having said this, each person's concussion and situation are different, and recovery will depend on a number of factors including whether they have other injuries or health issues.

Some people will be fine after a few days and able to return to life with relative ease while others will have a longer recovery journey. Take one day at a time, don't rush, develop self-awareness around your symptoms and triggers, pace yourself and trust your judgement as to how you feel and what your limitations are.

This sounds relatively straightforward but it can be quite hard to judge what you'll be able to do each day. You may find you tend to overdo things as you try to return to your pre-injury life. You might think you'll be able to do something but when you actually do it, it's a real struggle and then you end up crashing, sometimes for the best part of a day or for several days in a row.

While it's understandable and tempting to keep trying to push through and keep going at your pre-injury pace, in my experience it's not a good strategy and in the longer term, results in burnout. While it's good to challenge yourself to go to the next level or achieve the next goal, and while determination, persistence and perseverance are essential for recovery, pushing yourself too hard is counterproductive.

It really is a matter of trial and error because you can't know what you're capable of until you've tried to do something and know the outcome of doing it, which might be positive or negative. Over time, you'll get better at judging things. Be gracious, gentle and kind with yourself as you recover from a setback and don't let it stop you from keeping on trying in the future. Learn from the experience and make adjustments.

Brain fog and fatigue

Two common persistent symptoms after a concussion are brain fog and fatigue. There may be a number of contributing factors, some that occur earlier on post-injury and others that can develop over time, including:

- chronic inflammation in the brain as a result of the injury
- damage to neurons and axons
- disruption to various brain circuits and systems
- a reduction in blood flow in the brain
- changes in blood sugar levels
- mitochondrial dysfunction
- the brain having to work extra hard to do things, learn new things and rewire

- emotional issues – depression and anxiety – as part of the injury itself but also due to the way a person's life unfolds after injury and the added stresses and strains that causes
- dysregulation of the autonomic nervous system
- lack of exercise
- diet
- sleep disruption
- pain.

My own experience of fatigue after my concussion was feeling that I'd aged 40 years overnight. I frequently felt like I was swimming through treacle and I usually couldn't get through my day without taking a nap. Sometimes I slept all day, especially at weekends, having pushed myself too hard during the week. I'd have some good days but then I'd pay for it afterwards. Thankfully, I've learned many strategies for dealing with this, and although I still tend to tire more quickly, I'm better at managing my energy levels now. Below I share various strategies and techniques I've used to manage fatigue and overcome cognitive challenges that I hope you'll find helpful.

Spoon theory (fatigue management)

Spoon theory is a useful tool created by Lupus sufferer Christine Miserandino to help people understand and manage their energy levels. It illustrates how a healthy person starts the day with lots of energy and can go through their day relatively smoothly, without having to make too many choices about which activities to do. However, a person with a chronic health condition has limited energy levels and has to make choices about how they spend their energy, otherwise they will quickly end up feeling depleted.

Imagine you have 12 spoons per day and each spoon represents a unit of energy. Each task you do during the day is represented by a number of spoons. For example, eating breakfast or taking a shower might use up one spoon whereas driving, supermarket shopping or attending a doctor's appointment might use up three spoons. So, you may find that by a certain time of day you don't have many spoons left for the rest of the day. You then have to choose between activities in order to make the spoons last until the end of the day, based on how much energy you feel you have. So, you may have two spoons left which means you can cook dinner but then you have to choose between tidying your living room or spending time on a hobby. You can borrow spoons from the following day but then you will begin that day with a deficit, so there's a payoff for doing that. The aim is to try to learn how to make your spoons last longer so that you can manage your energy levels better.

Breathing exercises

Feeling anxious and frequently being in a state of 'fight or flight' can make your breathing shallower than usual. Doing breathing exercises regularly is a simple but surprisingly effective way to restore a sense of calm to yourself. You can do them several times a day, for a few minutes at a time, as and when you feel the need. I suggest you breathe in through your nose and out through your mouth. There are lots of different methods and exercises but below are some of the simplest:

1 Sit quietly somewhere and just breathe, focusing on every breath. If your breathing is fast, try to take longer breaths in and out, or a breath in and then a longer one out.
2 Breathe around an imaginary rectangle. Imagine a rectangle of any size in front of you. Take a deep breath in through your nose as you visualize one of the shorter lines of the rectangle. Then breathe out through your mouth as you imagine one

of the longer lines. Breathe in again as you picture the next shorter line and then breathe out again as you picture the next long line. Keep going a few times.

3 Breathe in for a count of six and then out for a count of ten. Repeat several times.

4 Breathe deeply in and out for a while and, as you do so, imagine yourself breathing in clean air and light and breathing out toxicity and darkness.

Mindfulness

Being mindful means being aware of the present moment, noticing how you're feeling and being fully engaged with what you're doing. Mindfulness helps you to anchor yourself in the present, rather than becoming caught up in the past or the future.

You can practise mindfulness by just sitting quietly in a chair or lying down or going for a walk and noticing what's around you. Look at your environment, notice what you see and hear and take everything in.

Mindfulness can be done at any time throughout the day too by paying close attention to what you're doing or noticing what's around you and applying it to all five senses. So, for example, if you're chopping vegetables then notice the vibrant colours, savour every mouthful of a delicious meal, take time to appreciate the beautiful smell of some flowers, enjoy listening to your favourite music or notice the sensation of touching a soft blanket.

Meditation

Meditation can calm your mind and help your body to get out of its 'fight or flight' sympathetic state into the 'rest and digest' parasympathetic state.

Here are some short instructions for a simple meditation:

1 Find a quiet spot and set a timer for about 10–15 minutes. At first you may only manage a minute or two. Any amount of time will do but keep trying every day or as often as possible and it will become easier.
2 Either sitting or lying down, preferably with your eyes closed, start to breathe in and out, taking long, deep breaths.
3 Focus on your breathing. If a thought comes into your head, then notice and acknowledge it but don't judge it. Don't get caught up in your thoughts; let them pass. Keep focusing back on your breathing.

There are apps like Calm and Headspace and lots of resources online, including free ones on YouTube, to help you with mindfulness and meditation. I also recommend Emily Fletcher's book *Stress Less, Accomplish More*.

Expanding the window of tolerance

Since my accident, I've often found it hard to stay within my 'window of tolerance'. This is a term developed by psychologist Dan Siegel to describe the emotional state in which a person functions at their best. There have been many times when I've experienced extremes of emotion. I've felt this either as intense anxiety and a flood of strong emotions (hyperarousal) or as being depressed, shut down and even dissociative (hypoarousal). For me, being within my window of tolerance is a sense that all is well with the world, and life is calm, connected and safe.

A concussion can cause disruption to the limbic system in the brain, the part that controls behaviours and emotions. Our brain's job is to keep us safe and it can interpret the injury as a threat to our safety. If this happens, the brain switches to high alert, constantly scanning the environment for danger. It can feel as if your danger alarm system (the amygdala, located in the limbic system) is permanently switched on and you may notice that you're hypervigilant, and feel almost constantly anxious, jumpy and on edge. This heightened sense of danger can be exacerbated by the injury itself, experiencing ongoing persistent symptoms as well as challenging life circumstances, for example trying to find the right medical support, losing a job or relationship difficulties.

I've used various tools and strategies within this chapter of the book to help me turn down the sensitivity of my internal alarm system. It takes a while to learn these strategies and put them into practice and you may find you need to frequently come back to them, but they can definitely help.

Learning how to regulate your autonomic nervous system

Therapist Deb Dana's book *Polyvagal Exercises for Safety and Connection* and her audio book 'Befriending Your Nervous System' are both excellent resources full of practical exercises for learning how to regulate your autonomic nervous system. Drawing on Stephen Porges's Polyvagal Theory – which asserts the important role of the vagus nerve in the function of the nervous system – Deb Dana identifies the three main 'vagal' circuits:

1 Ventral vagal – 'rest and digest': feeling calm, present and physically safe and emotionally connected to others.
2 Sympathetic – 'fight or flight': feeling angry, anxious, panicky, irritated.
3 Dorsal vagal – 'freeze': feeling shut down, withdrawn, dissociative and self-protective.

At any given time, depending on circumstances, a person's autonomic nervous system subconsciously moves them along a scale, through these various states, between a state of protection to one of safety, connection and social engagement.

Deb Dana explains how you can connect to and bring awareness to your autonomic nervous system and different bodily sensations through 'neuroception'. Neuroception is the way humans receive and interpret information from their inner state, the external environment and between the self and other people. Being curious about your autonomic nervous system and observing, without judgement, whether it's in a state of connection or protection helps you to feel more connected to your body, move between the different autonomic states with greater ease and become better at finding your way back to the ventral vagal state. My experience of having a brain injury is spending a lot of time in the sympathetic or dorsal state. Over time, I've learned to be able to go to the ventral vagal state more quickly and easily and I've become more emotionally and physically regulated and resilient.

Deb Dana says to imagine a line, with the three vagal states positioned along it, with ventral on the left, sympathetic in the middle and dorsal on the right. At any given moment, you can tune into where you are along that continuum. The more you become aware of where you are on that line, the easier it will be to change state. You can think of words, colours or music that describe your experience of being in each state. You can use activities, creativity, nature, people, music, memories, places and so on as 'anchors' to help bring you back into a ventral vagal state from the sympathetic and dorsal states. Many of the suggestions in this book can help you with this, for example moving, getting outside, journaling, using essential oils or spending time with a good friend. Experiment and find what works best for you.

The vagus nerve and increasing your vagal tone

The vagus nerve is the tenth cranial nerve, that wanders from the brain stem to the abdomen, carrying information between the brain and other organs in both directions. It plays a key role in activating the 'parasympathetic' or 'rest and digest' part of the nervous system, and affects your breathing, heart rate and digestive function.

I recommend the book, *Accessing the Healing Power of the Vagus Nerve* by Stanley Rosenberg. It's possible that a contributor to persistent concussion symptoms may be low vagal tone. In other words, the vagus nerve isn't functioning as well as it should, leading to a heightened stress response that can cause anxiety, depression, gut issues and inflammation. Increasing vagal tone helps the body to access its parasympathetic state and relax more quickly after stress. Activities which can help increase vagal tone include humming, singing, gargling and a number of simple exercises in Stanley Rosenberg's book. One of these exercises involves lying on your back with your legs straight and your hands placed behind your head. Lying in that position, you move your eyes to the left, while you keep your head straight, until you experience either a yawn or a sigh (usually between a few seconds and a minute), then you do the same on the other side. The yawn or sigh is a sign of increased vagal activity. You repeat this a few times up to several times a day.

Simple ways to restore a sense of safety to yourself

This section contains some simple ways you can move from feeling anxious to experiencing a sense of safety:

1 Gently put your hand on your chest or your stomach. Or give yourself a hug. Doing these simple things, and perhaps saying to yourself either internally or out loud, 'I'm OK, I'm safe', will tell your brain that things are fine and help to soothe you.

2 Dr Peter Levine, psychologist, trauma expert and developer of Somatic Experiencing, recommends making the sound

'Voo' out loud, in a low tone, and then repeating it several times, for 1–2 minutes. Then, observe how you feel for a minute or two. If you still feel tense then repeat the sound until you feel calmer. Alternatively, you could hum or make a different sound such as 'Aahh'.

3 Another of Levine's suggestions is to sit or lie in a quiet place, putting one hand on your forehead and the other one on your chest. After a short while, you can take the hand from your forehead and place it on your stomach and hold that position for a while. Notice how you feel. Alternatively, tuck your right hand under your left armpit and wrap the other arm around your stomach and hold that position for a while.

Both making the 'Voo' sound and holding any of these positions for a short while signals a sense of safety to your brain and body.

Harness the power of neuroplasticity

Neuroplasticity is one of the most powerful tools available to you as you recover from your concussion. Your brain is plastic, meaning it's malleable and can change. It's amazing that you can literally rewire your brain. The brain operates on the principle of 'Use it or lose it'. On the one hand, you can create new neural pathways or build up and strengthen existing ones. On the other, if you stop doing a certain activity or do less of it, the neural connections in your brain responsible for that become weaker and the activity becomes harder to do or you may forget how to do it.

Cognitive challenges after your concussion may have led you to believe that you are now intellectually inferior or stupid. That isn't the case at all. It's just that your brain's not working as efficiently as it previously did. It has to work harder and it takes longer for messages to travel along the neural pathways in the brain, due to either damage or disruption, so it takes longer to process things. Sometimes, it's more effective, rather than using the old path, to create a new one. The messages can start going down a newly forged narrow path that over time will become deeper and more well worn and eventually will turn into a superhighway that messages can run along quickly and efficiently.

I've read that it takes anything from 21 to 90 days to create a new neural pathway or a new habit. So, if you're trying to learn a new skill, way of thinking or way of doing something, then don't be discouraged if it's hard at first. Keep going because the more you do it, the easier it will get and eventually what seemed hard at first will become second nature.

Imagine a child learning to ride a bike or a person learning a musical instrument or a language from scratch. None of these new skills is picked up overnight. The person builds up gradually, adding layer upon layer of learning and practice, until they become proficient and finally reach mastery. This is the same with learning or relearning skills after a brain injury.

If you're struggling in a particular area, for example with walking, cooking, reading, writing or studying, then keep doing that activity over and over again, every single day. That's how I've approached my recovery. Gradually, you'll start to see improvements. Just keep going and keep trying. If something seems too hard then stop and rest or switch to doing something that isn't so taxing for a while and you can always come back to the skill you're working on another day. Or try doing the activity in a different way as the old way may not work so well. Most importantly, be patient. Think of a toddler learning to walk. They go from trying to stand to walking over a number of weeks and months. They repeat their actions over and over again and fall many times but they keep trying and eventually they get the hang of it.

Brain training

There are numerous ways you can retrain your brain and improve your cognitive abilities at home. A great starting point is the book *The Mild Traumatic Brain Injury Workbook* by Douglas J. Mason, which contains a variety of exercises to help you recover brain function.

Neuroscientist Donalee Markus has pencil and paper cognitive rehabilitation exercises available from her website <www.designsforstrongminds.com>, which are recommended by associate professor of artificial intelligence Clark Elliott in his book on his concussion, *The Ghost in My Brain*.

Doing puzzles, crosswords, quizzes and playing board games and computer games – including virtual reality – are all great for sharpening your mind.

There are conflicting views on whether tools such as brain-training apps and games are effective but personally, I've found them very helpful. Lumosity (<www.Lumosity.com>) is an excellent brain-training app that I'm sure helped me with cognitive skills such as working memory, mental flexibility, reaction times and word-finding. Games and training apps can improve certain specific skills and are transferable to real life, but real-life experiences are just as, if not more, important for rehabilitation.

I'm a big fan of online learning so I've taken a number of self-paced courses on Udemy on different subjects such as improving memory and speed reading. There's plenty of free information online but if you want more depth and application on a topic, I recommend taking a course.

Improving your memory

You may experience long-term and/or short-term memory problems after your concussion. I've experienced both, but thankfully things are better now for me than they were. Here are some things you can do to improve your memory:

- Use some of the strategies and techniques listed earlier in this chapter.
- Download and use the app Alfred, which has a 'smart prompt' for reminders as well as other useful rehabilitation resources. (Developed by Neumind, <www.neumind.com>, it's currently in Beta and available via the Apple App Store or Google Play Store by searching for 'Alfred ABI' or 'Neumind Alfred'.)
- Look back at photos, scrap books, books you've read, diaries and other reminders.
- Chat with family and friends about people, experiences and things you've done in the past.
- Watch films.
- Listen to music.
- Tap into emotions, especially pleasant ones, as you go about your daily life as this can bring back memories.
- Visit places you've been to before.
- Try using your sense of smell to trigger memories.
- Make associations and connections between words and create images and pictures in your mind of words or things you wish to remember so that you can recall them more easily. These can be really silly; the sillier the better as you will remember them more easily. For example, you want to remember to buy bananas, toothpaste and a notebook from the supermarket so picture a monkey eating a banana then brushing his teeth before writing in his notebook about how tasty the banana was.
- Read a book on memory improvement or take an online memory training course, for example on Udemy or Jim Kwik's 'Recall' class at <www.jimkwik.com>.

Developing organizational skills

Persistent symptoms after a concussion may include problems with attention, focus, memory and executive function. Below are some of the cognitive strategies I've implemented over time to help improve in all these areas and to become more organized. I learned these from various sources, including a six-week brain injury recovery course at my local Headway branch, two neuro occupational therapists, online groups, books, videos and courses. There are two main headings, 'Organizing your home life' and 'Organizing your work life', but there are crossovers between the two.

Don't feel you have to do all the suggestions and just pick a few every day that suit you and your personal circumstances, otherwise you'll feel overwhelmed. You may feel frustrated, having to relearn or reimplement things you used to do with ease and speed, but with persistent effort you'll find strategies that work for you. You'll be able to do certain tasks more consistently, easily and quickly and you'll probably have more energy too.

Organizing your home life

1   Create a timetable of your week. Have set times or days when you do certain tasks, such as washing, cleaning or admin. This builds predictability and certainty into your days. If you intentionally set a time to do a certain task, you're more likely to do it. Schedule everything, whether that's your household tasks, leisure activities, exercise, social media use, etc.
2   Write everything down to help you remember things.
3   Switch from using a month-to-view wall calendar to a day-per-page desk diary.
4   Create lists – either on paper, in an app such as Evernote or with a digital assistant. Have a daily to-do list, a weekly shopping list, a weekly meal planner and a list of less frequent tasks.

5   Use a large whiteboard so you can easily see what needs to be done.

6   Break down each task into small, manageable-sized chunks. Even if you do something for five minutes, like admin on the computer or tidying a part of your room, that's an achievement.

7   Alternate boring jobs with more fun activities so you feel more motivated.

8   Take frequent breaks. Reward yourself when you've achieved a task, no matter how small.

9   If you're OK using a computer then consider doing your shopping online as much as you can if you currently find going to the shops overwhelming.

10 Lower your standards and expectations. Perfectionism won't help your recovery.

11 Ask yourself if a task really needs to be done and whether it needs to be done right now. Can it wait? Could you drop it completely? Some things aren't actually that important and don't need doing anyway.

12 It doesn't matter if you don't achieve everything you set out to do in a day. Focus on what you did achieve. I have a saying that I still use: 'Less But Better.'

13 Keep your environment tidy, whether that's your desk, your bedroom or any room in your house. Put things away in the same place so you can find them. Keep your living space uncluttered. It may take time to achieve this so be patient with yourself.

14 Use a pill box with days of the week on so you can remember to take any daily medication or supplements you have.

15 Put up a sign in your kitchen or if you're working so others in your household can see you are busy and know not to interrupt you. At home, if you're working or busy focusing on a task, for example cooking, and you don't

want any distractions, put up a sign – for example, up a handwritten note saying 'Busy – Please Do Not Disturb' on a brightly coloured piece of paper – so that members of your household know you need to be left alone. This can be especially helpful if you have younger children.

16 Encourage people in your household to help you with chores. Accept help from friends and family.

17 If you can afford to have a cleaner or a gardener, even for just an hour or two a week, then consider hiring someone to help you so you can focus your energy on other things and on getting better.

Organizing your work life

If you're in the UK and you work for an employer then you're not obliged to tell them about your injury. However, in most cases it's probably beneficial to let them know, for various reasons. Your employer should make reasonable adjustments for you to continue your job. If possible, communicate with them about your struggles and difficulties and see if they can make accommodations for you. You may be able to negotiate a gradual return to work, fewer working hours, regular breaks, adaptations to your environment or a change in role. Unfortunately, not all employers are understanding of people who've experienced a brain injury. There are more details about returning to work after a brain injury on the Headway website (<www.headway. org.uk>), under '*Practical Issues, Returning to Work*'.

You may be able to return to your existing job after your injury or you may find it's not possible and you have to rethink what to do. You could work with a neuropsychologist to help you consider your future options.

Just a quick note on welfare benefits in the UK: if you're off work long term or out of work, then it's worth applying for benefits to give you some form of income. However, you may find that you don't qualify for them due to your symptoms and health struggles being hidden, not understood and not meeting the assessment criteria. For advice, speak to Headway or the Citizen's Advice Bureau. The charity Scope is currently working to create a fairer system of assessment for people with invisible health conditions.

Below are some tips for organizing your work life. Some of these are relevant for organizing your home life too and some of the suggestions in that section are relevant here.

1 Choose certain times of day when you know you have more energy to do certain tasks.
2 Build predictability and routines into your day and your week so you know what you're doing when.
3 Keep your workspace tidy and clutter-free. Have a place for everything so you can find the things you need easily. Keep information such as phone numbers and passwords in one place.
4 There are many different online tools you can use to organize yourself better, including Asana (for managing projects), Trello (an online Kanban board), Evernote (an app for note taking) and Otter (a speech to text app).
5 Focus on one thing at a time, rather than multi-tasking, so you don't get distracted. Every time you context switch and change task, you lose time because it takes about 20 minutes to get into a new task. Notice if your mind wanders off and bring it back.
6 Break tasks down into their most basic steps and do one step at a time.
7 As soon as you start to lose focus or feel fatigued, stop that activity and do something else. Aim to do something for 30 minutes if you can, but do less if that's all you can manage.
8 Take regular breaks in between tasks. Take as long as you need but gradually try to reduce those breaks if you can. If not, don't worry.

9   Learn to do things to the point that you don't bring on a flare-up of symptoms. Learn to know when to stop. In time, you'll get better at spotting the warning signs.

10 Learn to say no. Every time you say yes to something, you're saying no to lots of other things. People can't see what you have on your plate and it's easy to take on more and more. Be realistic about what you can and can't do and let your boss and co-workers know.

11 You'll feel more motivated and find it easier to focus if you enjoy what you're doing. Remind yourself regularly of what you enjoy about your job and why you're doing it.

12 Set yourself realistic expectations. Don't compare yourself to the people around you who haven't had a brain injury.

Operate in flow state

In life, we tend to mostly use the logical, reasoning part of our brain, which gives us that sense of pushing through and getting things done. Since my concussion, I've found this isn't always the best way to function as it contributes to the boom-and-bust cycle you may be familiar with.

I've learned to tap into a more intuitive, relaxed and creative way of operating much of the time, which takes the pressure off using the part of my brain which tends to go into overdrive and sometimes struggles with cognitive tasks. This could be described as 'being in flow'.

'Flow' is a state first identified by psychologists Mihaly Csikszentmihalyi and Jeanne Nakamura. It's a state where you feel focused, present in the moment, at one with the activity you're doing, unaware of time passing, at ease and more creative, imaginative and intuitive. In flow, you're operating not primarily from your logical mind, your prefrontal cortex, but rather from your subconscious mind. When in this state, different neurochemicals are released and different brain waves are activated, creating a positive feedback loop. It can be hard to activate this state initially, but I've found that through practices such as breathing, meditation and mindfulness, I've been able to access flow state more and more and now I can get into it and out of it with relative ease.

I've also had to learn to be OK with going at a gentler, slower pace than previously. Having to slow down can feel very frustrating initially. Over time, I've actually found some benefits to slowing down and I don't mind not racing about all over the place like I used to.

Develop self-awareness, change your thoughts and shift your emotional state

Self-awareness is the act of focusing attention on yourself in order to have a better understanding of yourself and how you relate to others and the world around you. As I became more self-aware, I started to see that I wasn't helpless and that to a degree I could change and choose my thoughts, which influenced how I felt emotionally, mentally and physically.

A person has thousands of thoughts every day. Your thoughts lead to certain emotions and actions that produce neurotransmitters which create different biochemical reactions in your body. Happy chemicals are manufactured in the brain when you engage in certain activities. For example, going for a run causes endorphins to be released, creating a positive feeling in your body; completing a task and rewarding yourself for doing so creates dopamine, which gives you a sense of accomplishment; remembering a happy time in the past creates serotonin, which lifts your mood; and sharing a meal with good friends produces oxytocin, which makes you feel connected. Conversely, worrying and feeling anxious all the time results in chemicals such as adrenaline and cortisol being released in your body. While these are helpful in the short term for escaping from a life-threatening situation, longer term they can lead to chronic stress and mental and physical health problems.

Post-concussion syndrome can go hand in hand with negative thinking. Psychiatrist Dr Daniel Amen calls automatic negative thoughts 'ANTs' and explains that initially these thoughts and emotions may have been trying to protect us and keep us safe but when we have an infestation of them, they become harmful and it's best to get rid of them.

Habitual negative thoughts are sometimes referred to as cognitive distortions. Although everyone has these to some degree, it's when they become fixed and unbalanced that they can cause problems. Some examples of cognitive distortions include black-and-white thinking, catastrophizing, overgeneralizing and focusing only on the negative aspects of life. Reducing our negative thinking restores balance to our mental, physical and emotional health.

By increasing your self-awareness, you'll be better able to identify if you're stuck in a negative-thought or emotional-feedback loop and work towards breaking it and changing your emotional state. Identifying and breaking out of negative patterns helps you to feel more positive and hopeful. You'll be better able to tune into your needs, wants and desires. You'll feel happier, make better decisions and gain clarity on how you want to move forwards in your life.

Below are some suggestions for changing your thoughts and shifting your emotional state:

1 Notice what you're thinking or feeling. Allow yourself to experience and feel your emotions and get curious about them. Ask yourself questions like, 'What emotion am I feeling here?', 'Why am I feeling like this?', 'Has something triggered me to feel like this?' and 'Is there a pattern here?' If you notice a thought or emotion that's unsettling you, then try to get to the root of it and take steps to address the issue. If you identify that you're stuck in a negative loop, then

make a decision to think or feel something different, possibly the exact opposite. You may want to write down or journal about the thoughts and emotions that come up for you in order to help you process them.

2 Bring awareness in your body to any emotion you feel, for example anxiety. Get curious about the feeling and notice where it's held: is it in your chest, stomach or somewhere else? How does it feel: is it tight, heavy or suffocating? Allow yourself to feel the emotion; don't push it away. Name the emotion. Label it, without judgement. The feeling may be so intense that you feel it could overwhelm you but it won't. You may feel emotional and want to cry. If that happens, go with it as the emotional release is healthy. The wave of intense emotion will pass and you will come out on the other side of it. According to neuroscientist Dr Jill Bolte Taylor, it takes approximately 90 seconds for an emotion to pass through your body. Once you've done this once or a few times, the power is removed from the sensation. You won't feel overwhelmed by it and you'll feel lighter and calmer. If you don't feel comfortable doing this yourself, then consider working with a therapist.

3 Notice how external circumstances and events affect you and contribute to how you're feeling emotionally, mentally and physically. Even seemingly small things can affect you quite deeply. Similarly, notice what's going on internally and observe how you respond to what's going on in your life. Notice if something in your life is affecting you negatively or positively and take action based upon that.

4 Focus on the positive. This isn't about false positivity, being unrealistic, ignoring your challenges or denying your difficulties. It's about choosing to look for the good things in your life in the midst of whatever you're going through. Every day positive things happen but we don't always appreciate them. Has a long-awaited medical appointment come through? Did you manage 10 minutes of an exercise routine? Did you go to

the supermarket without feeling dizzy? Did you make a tasty, healthy meal? Did your boss give you longer to work on a project? The more you focus on the positive things in your life, the more you will notice more of them and the happier you will feel.

5 Reframe your thoughts and choose to see things in a different light. An example from my life is that if I hadn't had my concussion, I wouldn't have given my diet an overhaul and I'd still be consuming way too much sugar and wouldn't be doing my health any favours.

6 Author Byron Katie has a simple short method of self-enquiry she calls 'The Work'. When a negative thought comes up, ask yourself if it's really true. So, for example, if you find yourself saying, 'I'm so useless', ask yourself, 'Is that true?' and then again, 'Is that really true?' If it isn't, then think of examples that provide evidence that it's not the case. Next, ask yourself how you feel when you think that negative thought. And then ask yourself how you would feel or who you would be without that thought. Notice any difference in how you feel as a result of going through this process.

7 If you find yourself feeling stuck and thinking you'll never get better, then when you notice that thought, determine to take an action instead that will shift your emotional state and help your recovery. For example, you may decide to do 10 minutes of yoga, go for a walk, do a creative activity or go to bed half an hour earlier.

8 Notice when you feel good and not just when you feel bad. What makes you feel happy, energized, excited or calm? Notice when you feel those things. Doing more of what you enjoy and what makes you feel happy will create more positive feelings and give you momentum for your recovery. So, for example, if you find that being in nature lifts your spirits, then do more of that. Keep engaging in activities that enhance your mental and physical well-being.

9 It can be helpful to use an app on your phone to record how you're feeling. Some apps I like for emotional and mental health and journaling are Remente, Mood Tracker Self-Care Balance, Prompted Journal and Three Good Things (from Plum Studio). They all have free versions on Google Play and the App Store. There are many others; just pick one or a few you like and find easy to use.

Processing your thoughts and emotions can be uncomfortable. You might be tempted to bury your feelings, push them away and generally avoid them. Strong emotions aren't necessarily 'bad'; they can be very important messages that alert us to something we need to give our attention to. It's what we do with those emotions that's important. It can be quite painful to allow yourself to feel and start to get curious and examine your emotions but you can build up gently and be compassionate with yourself. Your feelings and experiences can be great teachers. If you find it difficult to deal with and process your emotions, you may find it helpful to work with a therapist or counsellor.

Creating balance

Having persistent concussion symptoms can feel like being on a rollercoaster. Recovery isn't linear. You may have times when you're moving forwards and you feel pretty good and other times when you're making slow progress, no progress at all or you're going backwards, which can leave you feeling discouraged. It may seem that your whole life has been taken over by medical appointments and desperately trying everything to get better.

You need to keep going but you also need to remember that recovery takes time. Create balance by looking after yourself and doing things you enjoy, that help you relax and that give your life joy and meaning. It's good sometimes to just pull back and focus on other things, which I know is sometimes easier said than done. Below are some suggestions to help you create balance in your life.

Don't do too much all at once

When it comes to different therapies, treatments and strategies for managing symptoms and organizing and rebuilding your life, don't do too much at once. Just pick a few things you think will help you the most or that particularly resonate with you and try those for a while to see if they work. If you don't notice a change or seem to have reached a plateau, then stop for a while, try something new or swap things around on different days.

Journaling

Journaling helps you get your thoughts and feelings out of yourself and onto paper. I find the process of writing helps me to reflect on what's going well in my life and what isn't, identify where I'm stuck emotionally and notice where I need to do some inner work. Journaling has helped me focus on the next steps to take in my recovery and it has also been a tool to help me think about, plan and create my future.

You can use journaling to help you express yourself more fully; process emotions; overcome frustrations; develop empathy and compassion for yourself; outline goals and plans; and bring your dreams to life. You may find that having a regular journaling practice energizes you by freeing you up from thoughts and worries.

If you miss a day or stop for any reason, that's fine, don't be hard on yourself and just start again when you can. It doesn't have to be perfect; the main thing is to just do it. Start with about 5–15 minutes. You can keep what you write and re-read it straight away or at a later date, or you can throw it away.

There are a number of different ways you can journal; just do whatever works best for you. Here's a variety of suggestions:

1 The artist and writer Julia Cameron, author of *The Artist's Way*, recommends writing 'The Morning Pages' every day: three pages of stream-of-consciousness writing of whatever comes into your head to free up your mind as you start the day.
2 Check in with yourself. Write about specific emotions and feelings. Develop self-awareness through your writing.
3 Make a note of your stressors: both past stressors and ones in the present. Think and write about how you can address these.
4 Think about and plan the next steps of your recovery. Journal about what's working and what isn't and write about what changes you could make to whatever you're currently doing and what things you could try next.
5 Write down some things you're thankful for each day. You can write them down first thing in the morning or last thing at night.
6 Journal about your strengths and accomplishments throughout your life. Think back to times you've been coura-geous and strong, overcome hurdles and felt proud of what you've achieved. Remind yourself of what you're capable of.
7 Journal about your hopes and dreams and plan how you're going to get there.
8 Search online for different journal prompts and use those.

Core beliefs

Our beliefs extend beyond the spiritual dimension to how we see and relate to ourselves, others and the world. They come from our environment, inner thoughts, life experiences and upbringing. Over time, repetitive thoughts are laid down in our neural pathways and layers of beliefs are built up. We're always operating from our beliefs, rarely challenging or questioning them and often accepting them as part of our identity. For many of us, we think our thoughts and beliefs are who we are.

After my concussion, I felt like I'd partially lost my sense of identity. Not only did I feel like I was physically living in an alien's body that felt scary and unsafe, with unfamiliar sensations and symptoms, but, in many ways, I no longer felt like 'me'. My sense of who I was, my thoughts and some of my beliefs and how I saw the world seemed to have changed. This felt very unsettling; I had no compass for recovery, no blueprint for what I should do and no idea of what to expect. Nothing up to that point in my life had prepared me for the situation I now found myself in. I was in completely new territory.

As a result, some of the beliefs I'd previously had were no longer helpful in the new situation I found myself in and also, I was starting to subconsciously develop new beliefs. Some of these were helpful but others weren't at all. Let me give you an example of one of my limiting beliefs. For some time after my injury, I believed I was broken and beyond repair, not just physically but also cognitively and mentally. I worked on this with Dr Pradhan and I soon started to understand how my repeated thoughts were creating beliefs like this, which weren't serving me at all. I realized that if I changed my thoughts, I could create a new belief about my identity and after working this through, I was able to reframe how I saw myself. I was able to see that what I'd been through had actually made me stronger and taught me valuable life lessons that I could take with me into the future.

There are two beautiful Japanese concepts, 'Wabi-sabi' and 'Kintsugi', and these also helped me reframe my thoughts and beliefs about me being broken.

In a nutshell, Wabi-sabi is an artistic style, lifestyle and philosophy of authenticity, simplicity, transience and embracing imperfection. So, it's possible to appreciate, for example, dried flowers, a rusty gate, an asymmetric leaf or a favourite pair of well-worn slippers. I came to appreciate and value the messiness and rawness of my ongoing experience.

Kintsugi is the art of mending broken pottery with gold, the idea behind this being that the broken parts are worth keeping and are transformed into striking gold veins, representing resilience, strength and wisdom. These then become an integral part of the vessel, pointing to a story behind it and enhancing its quality and value.

Finally, I encourage you to find motivational quotes and affirmations or to create your own. Write them down or print them off and put them up somewhere you can see them in your house, by your desk or on your mobile phone. Look at them often and start to believe them for yourself. Our minds are powerful and they thrive on clarity, focus and direction. Make your mind your greatest ally in your brain recovery. Keep renewing your thoughts and beliefs and keep taking consistent action in order to achieve change. Below are some affirmations that you might like to use.

Affirmations for your concussion recovery journey

1 My brain is the most incredible supercomputer on Earth. I'm thankful for it.
2 I believe in myself and my ability to heal. I believe I can improve and make a good recovery.
3 I won't let anyone tell me I can't do something or anything stop me from making improvements.
4 Neuroplasticity – the brain's ability to change – is amazing. My brain has an incredible capacity to rewire and change. I can create new neural pathways in my brain that will help me to recover.

5   Neurogenesis–the brain's ability to regenerate–is extraordinary. My brain can grow new cells.

6   The concussion does not define me. I am not my concussion, just like I am not a broken leg or the flu.

7   I love my brain and I will do everything I can to create an optimal environment so that it has the best chance of recovery.

8   I will give myself grace and patience. I'm doing the best I can right now and that's more than good enough.

9   It's OK to slow down. In fact, slowing down when I need to will help me to heal. I may be able to accomplish less but I will do it better.

10   I am worthy of compassion, kindness, love and respect from myself and others.

11   I will give my time to activities, people, things and places that are life-giving and that support me and give me energy.

12   I am just as valuable a person on the tough days as on the good days.

13   I will take time to listen to my body, try to understand what it's telling me and respond accordingly.

14   I will build my mental and physical strength and pursue wellness.

15   If I have a setback, I know it will pass. I'm not stuck in that situation forever.

16   I am taking consistent action towards creating my best life possible.

Visualization

Visualization and guided imagery are great tools to have in your concussion recovery toolbox. Harnessing the power of your imagination can help you to shift into a different emotional state. Your brain doesn't always know the difference between what's real and what isn't, so when you imagine a beautiful calming scene, such as walking along a quiet beach with the waves lapping at your feet, your mind and body will respond as if you're actually there. You can feel calmer, happier and more courageous through visualization. You can even help shape your future using the power of your imagination. This can all have a positive effect on your physiology. There are many different strategies and resources available, including YouTube videos, on visualization. I'll share a few different simple techniques below. They can take just a few minutes or longer and can be done lying or sitting down in a quiet place, with or without calming music. Practise visualization regularly.

1 Imagine being in a scene in nature such as a beach, a forest with a waterfall or on a snow-capped mountain. Create the scene in great detail in your imagination. Notice any changes in your mind and body as you explore the scene.

2 Picture yourself as your ideal self in the future, healed and well. What do you look like? How do you feel? Who are you with? What are you doing?

3 Bring to mind a situation that is weighing on you. You probably see it as large and overwhelming. Start to shrink it down and see it moving away from you towards the horizon, getting smaller and smaller until it disappears. You may notice that as you do this, the negative emotions attached to the situation lessen. You can stop there, or if you wish, you can then try the following. Think of a situation that makes you feel happy. Picture that far off in the distance and then bring it towards you so that it gets bigger and bigger. Notice and allow yourself to experience the associated thoughts and feelings that go with the scene.

4 The 'golden ball' visualization is a popular one. Imagine a golden ball of light slowly moving throughout your body

and brain. As it travels from your feet up to your head, or from your heart radiating out to your outer extremities, imagine it removing any blocks or impurities. Imagine your body being flooded with light. Imagine the ball then coming out of the top of your head and going up into the sky far, far away into the outer reaches of the universe. Imagine it coming back into your body and filling you with light again.

5 Imagine a large strong magnet, surrounded with a ring of fire, a metre or so in front of your body. Picture the magnet attracting negative thoughts and emotions, anxiety, limiting beliefs, worries, bad experiences and so on from you. As these leave you and attach to the magnet, they're burned up by the fire. Then imagine the magnet at your back and repeat the process and, if you wish, you can do the same down your sides and above your head and below your feet. (From the book *Recover Your Energy* by Olive Hickmott, 2009.)

Self-care

Make self-care a priority. Part of the process of regaining your confidence after a concussion is making it a priority to look after yourself. Self-care isn't frivolous and it doesn't have to be onerous. Make small changes every day and these will build up to make noticeable improvements in your health and well-being. Self-care looks different for each person but here are some things you could try:

1 Listen to your favourite music.
2 Listen to binaural beats. You can find these for free on YouTube. They are particular frequencies of sounds that are said to affect our brain waves and our mood. They may also help to relieve anxiety or create focus.
3 Listen to an audiobook or podcast.
4 Make healthy lifestyle choices and make time to implement them.

5   Celebrate small wins. It doesn't matter how big or small, every win you have is worth celebrating. This will release brain chemicals that make you feel good and motivate you to keep going.

6   The words you say to yourself are important, so speak to yourself using affirming, compassionate, forgiving, gentle, kind, non-judgemental, non-critical language.

7   Spend time on hobbies and creative activities.

8   Learn something new, for example a language or cooking new recipes, because this will create new neural connections in your brain. Benefits include better attention, memory and problem-solving skills.

9   Read books about or watch films, documentaries and YouTube talks on topics you're interested in, and especially by and about inspirational people.

10 Build happy, fulfilling moments into your day, taking time here and there to do things you really enjoy and that help you feel secure and happy.

11 Have realistic expectations and don't be hard on yourself. At the end of the day, know you've done your best.

12 Wind down with a relaxing bath at the end of the day, maybe with some essential oils, bubble bath or Epsom salts.

13 Make the most of your time away if you go on holiday. Your healing accelerates when you're in a relaxed state. Be aware that packing and the journey may be challenging but you should still be able to enjoy your time away.

Essential oils

Essential oils have many benefits, including subtly altering mood and relieving symptoms such as tension and headaches. Use essential oils with an electric essential oil diffuser, put a few drops into a roller ball with a carrier oil such as grapeseed or coconut oil or add a few drops into a carrier oil and add to a warm bath. I have a wonderful sleep spray from Tisserand which contains essential oils such as lavender and jasmine. I recommend the book *Essential Oils, Ancient Medicine* by Dr Josh Axe.

Some of my favourite oils include:

- frankincense for calm and focus
- lavender to calm you and help you sleep
- bergamot, lemon and orange for clarity and to lift your mood
- peppermint and rosemary for headaches
- rosemary to help with focus and attention.

Spend time outdoors in nature

Spending time outdoors in natural surroundings helps you relax and reset, whether it's going for a walk in the park, the woods or along a beach. It's a great opportunity to leave your worries behind and focus on the here and now. Listen to the sounds of the birds, the wind in the trees and the leaves scrunching under your feet; breathe in the fresh air and take in the sights, smells and sounds around you. Your head will feel clearer and you'll feel more energized and alive. Being out in sunlight tops up your vitamin D levels and increases melatonin, which helps with sleep.

Gratitude

Expressing gratitude helps to rewire the brain into a more positive mindset. It's such a simple, yet powerful, thing to do, especially once it becomes a regular habit. Start and end your day thinking about or writing down several things you're thankful for. Or make a mental note of what you're grateful for as you go through your day.

Laughter

I lost my sense of humour for a couple of months after my accident and there have been plenty of times over the last few years when laughing hasn't been at the top of my priority list. Recovery can be a very serious business and rightly so at times, but it doesn't have to be all the time. The saying goes that laughter is the best medicine and there's a lot of truth in that. Even when things are tough, it can be a real tonic to laugh sometimes and see the funny side of life. Watch some funny movies, read a funny book or enjoy a laugh with family or friends. Incorporate some fun into your days and cultivate a curious, playful attitude to life.

Spirituality and faith

Having persistent symptoms after a concussion can affect the very core of your being. You may feel as if your beliefs, values and many of the things that make you who you are have been shaken.

You may have found this applies to your spiritual life, if you identify as a spiritual person. Spirituality can be affected by a head injury. For years, scientists have been investigating the brain to see if they can find a section that creates and controls our spiritual side. They've found certain circuits in the brain and associated neural processes they believe to be involved in the human experience of spirituality. It's certainly possible that these circuits are affected by a brain injury, changing our spiritual perception.

Aside from this, if you're a spiritual person then your injury and the ensuing course your life has taken may have made you question your faith. You may have asked yourself questions such as, 'Why didn't I do something to stop this happening to me?',

'How could God allow this to happen to me?' and 'Why am I suffering like this?'

At times, I've felt angry and abandoned by God and I've questioned my beliefs. I've been a Christian for many years but my injury rocked my faith. Not only did I question the benevolent nature of a good god, but at church, I found it difficult to sit still and concentrate during services due to symptoms such as pain, dizziness and noise and light sensitivity and at home I struggled to concentrate on spiritual practices.

Over time, I've processed and worked through what has happened to me and I've come to view things in a different light. I can now see that my faith helped to give me hope and strength to keep going even when things were at their most difficult. I've also felt very blessed by kindness from people, whether friends, family, healthcare providers or strangers. Over time, as my symptoms have improved, I've been able to re-develop a spiritual practice and my faith has remained intact.

If you do have a faith but you feel as if your injury has impacted it, then either now or at a later time, you might want to start spending some time nurturing your spiritual life again and seeking answers to the questions you may have. You can do this in various ways such as reading books, meditating on uplifting quotes, spending time in meditation, prayer or reflection, journaling or talking to someone in your faith community about what you're going through.

For me, a key shift in my beliefs has been going from feeling that I've been punished to accepting that I'm loved by God or the universe, no matter whether I'm having a good or a bad day. It doesn't matter whether you have a faith or not, the important thing is to remember that you're a person of value and worth. Your value is not tied up in who you are on your best days; your value is the same, no matter what kind of a day you're having and no matter what you do or don't achieve.

Social relationships and seeking support

Spend time with the people you care about and who care about you; who you can be yourself with; who you're happy to be around and who support you and lift you up. Stay connected with people as much as possible and don't hide away or think you're a burden.

Be open with the supportive people in your life, whether that's certain family members, friends or neighbours, about how you're feeling so they can better understand what you're going through. You may need assistance with practical tasks such as grocery shopping, cooking or the school run, so just ask. Reach out to others for help; don't try to do everything yourself.

If you have children, you're still their parent. They still love, need and want to be with you. Don't worry about not being a 'good enough' parent. My children have been non-judgemental, forgiving and accepting of me throughout my recovery, even when I've felt at my very worst. I love and appreciate them so much for that. If you need help looking after your children at any time, then accept any offers from friends and family.

Be present and connect with the people you live with. This might seem a strange thing to say but there may be times when you have to remind yourself to do this. After your concussion, you may experience dissociation or a feeling of zoning out from your surroundings. This may be due to a number of factors, including fatigue, pain, emotional upset and as a direct result of your injury. Just noticing if you're doing this can be enough to act as a reminder to intentionally be more present. You can also make yourself start a conversation, for example, or you can ground yourself by noticing and focusing on certain things in your environment. Both of these can help to bring you into the here and now. Even if you feel you aren't joining in with conversations and activities as you used to, the people who care about you will appreciate your presence, interactions and contributions.

When it comes to social situations, there are plenty of things you can do to make things go more smoothly. Imagine you're meeting a friend at a café. First of all, choose a quiet spot to sit in that isn't too bright or noisy. You can explain to your friend that you're experiencing some difficulties and you should be fine but you may, for example, have to ask them to speak more slowly. You don't always have to mention your concussion or that you're struggling but there are definitely times when it's a good idea to. Bring your full attention to the moment and focus closely on your friend speaking, making regular eye contact. You may need to concentrate very hard on what they're saying and actively work to block out the distractions around you. During the conversation, ask questions and make comments and you can mirror back things that your friend has said, especially important things you want to remember. Remember to ask them questions too and don't just talk about yourself. It's fine to ask them to slow down so you can better follow what they're saying. If you're in a group, you may find it easier to just speak to one person at a time. And if you need to, you can always take a short break, find a quieter spot or look out of the window. You may want to have in mind a time limit for the meetup so you don't go beyond your limitations and start feeling symptomatic. It's fine to leave early or cancel beforehand if you don't feel up to it. If you find it's too much to go out to meet someone, then invite them over to your house instead or arrange to meet up somewhere quiet, like a park.

If you don't feel like meeting up in person, then stay in touch online on Zoom, WhatsApp, Messenger or by phone. You can have the screen switched on or off, depending on how you feel.

When you feel ready, do reach out to others. Remember, you're still a friend to people and can help them too, if they need it, either in practical ways or just by having a chat or listening. This goes for people in your immediate circle or others in your community or online. Don't feel helpless and powerless or think that you have nothing to offer because of your injury and symptoms. We all have something to give, no matter what our circumstances are. Even just sending a reassuring text to a friend, having a WhatsApp video chat or inviting someone round to catch up can mean a lot.

You may find that while some people are kind, understanding and willing to help you, some aren't so empathic and others may completely disappear from your life. The reality is that brain injury is poorly understood in our society. There may be people you know who simply cannot understand what has happened to you, and their way of coping may be to either pretend nothing has happened, blame you, ignore you or tell you you're making things up, which can be very upsetting. Some people just don't have the bandwidth, knowledge or inner resources to know how to relate to someone with a brain injury. While this doesn't excuse people, I hope it helps you to not take people's negative reactions to you so personally. It's important to protect yourself and have boundaries, so limit the time you spend with those who don't support you and focus on the people who do.

If you find yourself struggling emotionally, then do let people know. If you need someone to talk to outside of your immediate circle, or you need information on brain injury, there's the helpline of the brain injury charity Headway in the UK (tel: 0808 800 2244). Most regions in the UK have a local Headway group which may be able to help in a number of ways. Similar organizations exist in different countries. If you're in the UK and you're feeling truly overwhelmed and don't know where else to turn then you can call the Samaritans on 116 123. They will always lend a non-judgemental, sympathetic ear even if you're not feeling suicidal. There's also Shout, the UK's text crisis line, which you can text on 85258. Longer term, perhaps think about speaking to a counsellor, neuropsychologist or therapist.

Be inspired by others

Be inspired. Seek out inspiring and positive stories of people who have overcome different obstacles in life. Read books about inspiring people. Listen to podcasts and read blogs and articles about other concussion and brain injury survivors who have overcome their difficulties and are doing well. You'll glean lots of useful information, ideas and insights from them and see what it's possible to achieve. If others can make a good recovery, you can too. At the same time, don't compare yourself and your situation directly as you're on your own healing path and it will look different from that of other people.

Pets and animals

Pets and animals can be very therapeutic as you know if you have any pets. If you don't have your own pet, maybe you can ask a neighbour or friend to bring over theirs for a while or you could visit someone with one. Alternatively, you could take a trip to a local farm or zoo. This may be for further along on your recovery journey but it's something you could do when you're able to.

10

Moving forwards rather than looking back

Some people only have symptoms for a few days or weeks after their concussion and then they're able to return to normal life relatively easily. For other people, it takes longer; for some, months and for others, years, and life might look different from how it used to. Both of us, from a professional and an expert-by-experience perspective, believe it's possible, with the right help and tools, to make progress and a good recovery at any time after a concussion.

One of the most helpful lessons I (Anna) learned on my healing journey is that recovery from a brain injury is shaped like a 'W' and not like a 'Y'. A lovely counsellor at my local Headway branch shared this illustration with me. After a brain injury, a person wants to return to how they and their life were before. This is represented by the top part of the 'Y', moving from the top-right backwards to the top-left point. The pull to return to how things were is very strong, and many people find themselves intensely focused on wanting to go back to exactly how their life was. As long as a person remains in that position, they're likely to experience feelings such as anger, anxiety, despair, frustration and sadness. It can be very freeing to learn that brain injury recovery is actually shaped like a 'W'. In other words, if you start at the top-left hand of the 'W' and work down, then go up and down and up again, you will see that there will be ups and downs along the journey but the general direction is forwards.

Acceptance

This journey forwards may involve going through a period of mourning and loss for what was. If you experience that, then it's completely understandable and you're not alone; many people go through it. The enormity of the implications, consequences and knock-on effects of the injury can at times feel overwhelming.

You can't go back and change the past but you can process your emotions and work through what has happened to you in order to shape and create a fulfilling life and a meaningful future, whether you're fully healed or not. There is hope and you can determine to make the most of the rest of your life. You might find it helpful to work with a counsellor, coach or therapist to help you move forwards.

'Acceptance' means acknowledging your difficulties and challenges but choosing to carry on as best you can in spite of them. Reaching a point of acceptance is a process and it takes a different length of time for each person to get there. It's really important, as you recover, to treat yourself with compassion and forgiveness and without judgement.

Forgiveness

You may need to forgive yourself for sustaining your injury, a person or people who injured you, or people for misunderstanding or mistreating you. Forgiveness doesn't condone or excuse a person's actions but it does free you from heavy, overwhelming thoughts and feelings such as anger and resentment. Ultimately it will bring you peace and help you to move on. Forgiveness can only happen when you are ready and it's a process for each person. It takes time and there are no shortcuts to it. You may wish to seek professional help with this.

Why do some people recover and some people have persisting symptoms?

Below are some of the main factors that I think can contribute to some people taking longer to recover from persistent concussion symptoms than others. These points are based on my personal experience and research as well as the experiences of numerous people with post-concussion syndrome I've heard from in both the UK and worldwide.

- The severity of the injury.
- The extent of and number of symptoms a person has.
- Whether the person sustained any other injuries at the time of their concussion, for example a neck injury, fractures or whiplash.
- The age and sex of the person. For example, research indicates that older people and women are more prone to experiencing persistent symptoms.
- Whether a person has other pre-existing physical or mental health conditions, including previous head injuries.
- Whether the concussion has caused hormonal imbalances.
- Whether the person develops PTSD from their injury or whether they had pre-existing trauma from previous life experiences.
- The wide prevalence of misdiagnosis. Sadly, some people are even told they're making up their symptoms. If misdiagnosis occurs, it can take a long time to get a proper diagnosis and effective treatment.
- Lack of proper assessment early on after the injury.
- Difficulty finding information, knowledgeable healthcare providers and effective treatments and self-management solutions for the multiple facets of recovery – cognitive, emotional, mental and physical – and the challenges of doing that while experiencing brain injury symptoms.

- Whether a person is open to trying different treatments and modalities, including alternative, natural and innovative methods.
- A person's overall lifestyle.
- How well a person is able to learn to pace themselves.
- Whether a person takes an active or passive role in their recovery.
- To what extent the person has a supportive network of family and friends.
- The general lack of education, knowledge and understanding around brain injury among society in general, including the education, medical and legal sectors and in the workplace, which can lead to misunderstandings and a lack of support.
- Being involved in a legal case or making an insurance claim, which can add extra stress, complications and contribute to a prolonged recovery.
- The financial means of the person and what treatment they can afford or what treatments will be covered by medical insurance.
- What treatments are available to them near to where they live.
- The extent of the impact of the injury on a person's life – for example, whether they end up losing their job, a relationship, their home, etc.
- Whether a person already had some challenging life circumstances to deal with at the time of their injury.

Below are some proposals I believe would significantly improve the outcomes for people suffering from persistent concussion symptoms. Some of these points were suggested by fellow concussion survivors I was in contact with on social media.

- Having an early, comprehensive, detailed medical evaluation.
- Having timely access to treatment.
- Having a clear, holistic and multifaceted care pathway, addressing the physical, cognitive, mental and emotional

aspects of recovery and tailored to the needs of the individual.

- Better coordination between all the different branches of healthcare involved in a person's recovery; being assigned a case manager would help with this.
- Having more advocates who can speak up for and on behalf of patients.
- More alternative, holistic and personalized treatments available via a person's health insurance.
- Having better access to disability benefits and proper assessment by trained personnel.
- Education for the patient on self-management techniques alongside health treatments and therapies; provision to patients of healthy brain and lifestyle advice by doctors and other healthcare providers.
- Greater education and awareness of concussion and brain injury and its effects among doctors, healthcare professionals, A&E departments, the legal profession, employers, schools, sports coaches, etc.
- Greater awareness among the general population of concussion and brain injury which would hopefully lead to a better understanding of people who've had a brain injury.

Focusing on the future

I'd just like to share with you some aspects to focus on as you move forwards with your life:

1 Continue to have dreams and hopes for your future. You can journal about them if you like. Your dreams and hopes will keep you going, even when things in the present are tough.
2 Connect to your why and your purpose and let these guide you.
3 Identify your values and incorporate these into your daily life and your vision for your future.

4 Note down your achievements, attributes, skills, strengths and passions. Be intentional about how you want to spend the rest of your life.

5 Set yourself clear, measurable, achievable goals and take consistent steps towards them.

6 Spend time on personal development and growth work.

7 Identify any good things that have come out of your experience. For me, two good things have been learning to live a healthier lifestyle and developing an interest in all things brain-related.

There's strength in your weakness and you can turn your pain and struggles into something that can make a difference to others. What you've been through hasn't been wasted. You may at some point want to reach out to others and share your experiences, for example through local support groups, charities, with a blog or via social media. Research shows that helping others not only has obvious benefits for the recipients but has health benefits for the helper, including building confidence and self-esteem. And if you don't wish to do any of that then you may be surprised to find that you develop qualities of resilience and strength that positively influence others more than you realize.

Post-injury growth

I want to share with you a picture of what it has felt like for me trying to rebuild my life after my concussion. Maybe you can relate to this too.

Imagine that your house has been destroyed due to a natural disaster. Some rooms remain standing, some have disappeared altogether, and others have been left half-demolished, as smouldering shells of their former selves. Pictures have fallen off the walls, furniture has been smashed, rubble is piled high, and the scene is one of general devastation. You feel paralyzed by the scene in front of you.

After getting over the initial shock, disbelief and sadness, you walk slowly through the house, surveying the scene, taking it all in and wondering what on earth you're going to do about it.

You decide to set about restoring the house over the next few months. You clear away the rubble and debris and start to look at possibilities for renovation and repair. You realize that some rooms don't actually need too much doing to them. You dust them down, clean them, give them a coat of paint and rehang the pictures. Where there's greater damage, you decide to knock down certain rooms and start to rebuild them from scratch. To be honest, you tell yourself, you never did much like that kitchen anyway; the décor was a bit outdated. You're surprised that you start to feel happy that you have a chance to redo it with a nice, clean, modern look. Things are starting to look a lot better. You think to yourself, 'That dining room extension I always wanted but never got round to building, well, I'm going to invest in and build that now, rather than waiting any longer.'

After many months of rebuilding, extending, redecorating and renovating, you now have a beautiful house, and there are some parts that are even better than before. Sure, there are still reminders of the damage: a few cracks in the wall here and there and a few places where you can see the joins between the older and newer parts. Every now and again there's a maintenance problem, such as the roof leaking or an issue with the electrics, which needs some attention. Overall, though, you're satisfied with the finished result, you've learned a lot of useful lessons and skills along the way, and this house will serve you well now and into the future.

So, what does this image of the house have to do with post-injury growth? Think of the house as your life after your concussion. With the right help, rehabilitation, resources, determination, focus and encouragement, it's possible to make a good recovery. You've survived and now you can heal, transform and come out of the experience stronger and wiser.

For me, growth has meant, among other things: developing an empathy for others who have been through a similar experience; learning to appreciate the simple things in life; developing a greater appreciation of my husband and three children; challenging myself and trying new things; meeting new people; investing time in personal development and forging a new path as a writer, coach and advocate for concussion.

I have a desire to seize opportunities in life and make the most of every day. I don't want to waste time. I feel more focused on what I want to achieve with the rest of my life. I'm proud of myself for getting through these trials and overcoming a very difficult situation. I still face challenges every day and still have a way to go but I don't want to let my limitations stop me. I wish the same for you.

You may have to choose a different path. Your life may unfold in a way you never planned for. You may have to make certain changes in your life. This can be frustrating and upsetting but on the other side of it you will discover new facets of yourself, new experiences and new opportunities.

For a long time, I felt like a failure. I wasn't sure if I'd be able to work again. At the time of my accident, I was a full-time mum to three young children and I had to pull back from a lot of the things we did as a family and switch to different ways of doing life. Thankfully, I was able to continue to look after them with help from friends and family, although there were many times I felt like a terrible mother. Many aspects of life, including many plans and dreams for the future, went on the back burner.

Thanks to the neuropsychological work I did with Dr Pradhan, all the other help I had from healthcare and other professionals, and the support I had from my husband, children, friends and others, I was able to regain a lot of my skills and functionality and I found a sense of purpose again.

I began to wonder how I could bring good out of a bad situation and use what I'd been through to help other people. I thought about my career history in areas including counselling, business and publishing and I wondered how I could integrate those with my more recent life-changing experiences. I reflected on what aspects lit me up and what I thought I could still do as well as what I'd struggle to do. I spent time journaling about my dreams and drew a mind map of my skills, strengths and attributes. I did a lot of soul-searching and undertook some personal development work. Today, my main focus is still my family but I've gradually been able to develop other areas of my life. I've been able to forge a new path for myself. Over the past two years, I've done life coaching training, taken an online business course, written blog articles on concussion recovery, raised awareness of concussion and brain health, and now I've written this book.

I've learned that so much can be achieved by believing, searching, experimenting, making changes, keeping going and not giving up. I hold onto life coach Marie Forleo's mantra: 'Everything is Figureoutable'; yes, even something as complex as concussion recovery. There are still some things I find difficult to do and I still get flare-ups of symptoms, but I'm determined to not let that stop me from living my best life possible.

Keep going and don't give up

I've continued to heal though I still have a way to go. Sometimes I feel completely normal and other times I have quite significant flare-ups of symptoms. There are certain things that I find require more effort, especially some cognitive tasks such as planning and writing. I have less mental flexibility than I used to, find it harder to manage multiple tasks, tire more quickly and take longer to do certain things than I previously would have done. Overall, though, I do continue to make progress. I believe that no matter what your diagnosis is and no matter how much time has passed since your injury, there's always hope and room for improvement.

Even when you're moving forwards in your life, you may find yourself looking back from time to time, and that's OK. While it's good every now and again to remind yourself how far you've come, it's important to keep making the most of the here and now and to keep pressing on.

You may reach a plateau and think, 'That's it, I'm not going to recover any more.' You might think that's where you're going to stay. You may find yourself getting discouraged, coasting or feeling resigned, not realizing that you can make further improvements. If that happens, don't forget that your brain is extraordinary, and not only can it rewire and regenerate but parts of it can take over from other parts that are functioning sub-optimally. Sometimes, when you don't feel as if you're making progress, things are actually happening behind the scenes and beyond your awareness but you may only experience the results later on.

Do keep going, and don't give up. Recovery and change take time. Sometimes change is dramatic and other times it's slow and steady. While you'll want to be proactive and take consistent action, you can't rush recovery, so give yourself a lot of grace. You are developing resilience as you go. Be courageous, patient, persistent and determined. Determination is probably the main characteristic that has got me to where I am today.

Final thoughts

People are often surprised to learn that a 'mild' brain injury can cause such a wide range of symptoms with far-reaching effects on a person's life. The human brain is the most complex super-computer on Earth yet it has a similar consistency to jelly or tofu, making it delicate and vulnerable to strong blows and forces. The brain is the control centre of every part of a person's life. It not only keeps us alive but also plays a central role in our beliefs, emotions, intelligence, memories, movement, speech, thoughts and more. So, when the brain gets injured and as a result doesn't work as it should, it's understandable that various aspects of a person's being can be affected.

Concussion is not for the faint-hearted. There is no magic pill or single miracle cure for long-term concussion symptoms, but be encouraged: with the right medical help, information, outlook, tools and practice it IS possible to make a good recovery after a concussion. It's important to note that every person is unique and each brain injury is different, so the degree of improvement will depend on a number of factors relating to the individual person, the nature of their injury and the treatment and rehabilitation they receive. Some people will recover in a few days while others will take much longer.

Recovery may not be easy but it's doable and it's the little steps that make the difference. Thanks to neuroplasticity, our brains are adaptable and can change, even after an injury, so there's scope for the brain to rewire itself and heal. This offers hope to those who sustain a brain injury, to caregivers of someone who has and to those who treat patients.

Determine to live your healthiest possible life from now on and to take an active, rather than a passive, role in your healing. An important part of recovery is educating yourself about the brain and how it works and learning about brain health and the many different treatment options available. Seek out the people and resources that can help you. Keep pushing doors, putting one foot in front of the other, making small incremental changes and putting into practice what you learn. You also need to believe that recovery is possible. Don't give up. You can improve from where you are now.

References

Allder, S. & MacSweeney, E. (2021). *Recent Developments in neuro-imaging for traumatic brain injury*. Journal of Personal Injury Law.

American Psychiatric Association (2013). *Diagnostic and statistical manual of mental disorders: DSM-5* (5th ed.). American Psychiatric Publishing.

Bègue, I., Adams, C., Stone, J., & Perez, D. L. (2019). Structural alterations in functional neurological disorder and related conditions: a software and hardware problem? *NeuroImage: Clinical*, 22, 101798. https://doi.org/10.1016/j.nicl.2019.101798

Biagianti, B., Stocchetti, N., Brambilla, P., & Van Vleet, T. (2020). Brain dysfunction underlying prolonged post-concussive syndrome: A systematic review. *Journal of Affective Disorders*, 262, 71–76. https://doi.org/10.1016/j.jad.2019.10.058

Caplain, S., Chenuc, G., Blancho, S., Marque, S., & Aghakhani, N. (2019). Efficacy of Psychoeducation and Cognitive Rehabilitation After Mild Traumatic Brain Injury for Preventing Post-concussional Syndrome in Individuals With High Risk of Poor Prognosis: A Randomized Clinical Trial. *Frontiers in Neurology*, 10, 929. https://doi.org/10.3389/fneur.2019.00929

Diez, I., Williams, B., Kubicki, M. R., Makris, N., & Perez, D. L. (2021). Reduced limbic microstructural integrity in functional neurological disorder. *Psychological Medicine*, *51*(3), 485–493. https://doi.org/10.1017/S0033291719003386

Malec, J. F., Brown, A. W., Leibson, C. L., Flaada, J. T., Mandrekar, J. N., Diehl, N. N., & Perkins, P. K. (2007). The mayo classification system for traumatic brain injury severity. *Journal of Neurotrauma*, *24*(9), 1417–1424. https://doi.org/10.1089/neu.2006.0245

National Academies of Sciences, Engineering, and Medicine; Health and Medicine Division; Board on Health Care Services; Board on Health Sciences Policy; Committee on Accelerating Progress in Traumatic Brain Injury Research and Care, Matney, C., Bowman, K., & Berwick, D. (Eds.). (2022). *Traumatic Brain Injury: A Roadmap for Accelerating Progress*. National Academies Press.

Nelson, L. D., Temkin, N. R., Dikmen, S., Barber, J., Giacino, J. T., Yuh, E., Levin, H. S., McCrea, M. A., Stein, M. B., Mukherjee, P., Okonkwo, D. O., Robertson, C. S., Diaz-Arrastia, R., Manley, G. T., and the TRACK-TBI Investigators, Adeoye, O., Badjatia, N., Boase, K., Bodien, Y., Bullock, M. R., … Zafonte, R. (2019). Recovery After Mild Traumatic Brain Injury in Patients Presenting to US Level I Trauma Centers: A Transforming Research and Clinical Knowledge in Traumatic Brain Injury (TRACK-TBI) Study. *JAMA Neurology*, *76*(9), 1049–1059. https://doi.org/10.1001/jamaneurol.2019.1313

Prince, C., & Bruhns, M. E. (2017). Evaluation and Treatment of Mild Traumatic Brain Injury: The Role of Neuropsychology. *Brain Sciences*, *7*(8), 105. https://doi.org/10.3390/brainsci7080105

Sharp, D. J., & Jenkins, P. O. (2015). Concussion is confusing us all. *Practical Neurology*, *15*(3), 172–186. https://doi.org/10.1136/practneurol-2015-001087

Smith, D. H., & Stewart, W. (2020). 'Concussion' is not a true diagnosis. *Nature Reviews Neurology*, *16*(9), 457–458. https://doi.org/10.1038/s41582-020-0382-y

World Health Organization. (2004). *ICD-10: international statistical classification of diseases and related health problems* (tenth revision, 2nd ed.). World Health Organization. https://apps.who.int/iris/handle/10665/42980

Resources and further reading

Concussion Recovery

Blaskovich, S., & O'Brien, E. (2020). *Dr B's concussion breakthrough: Exploring the hidden connection to neck injuries and a simple guide to naturally heal your brain.* [Self-published].

Bottomley, D. (Host). *Post-Concussion Syndrome Awareness Podcast.* [Audio podcast].

Chapek, K. (2020). *Concussion rescue: A comprehensive program to heal traumatic brain injury.* Citadel Press.

Chiu, T. (2018). *BrainSAVE: The 6-week plan to heal your brain from concussion, brain injuries & trauma without drugs or surgery.* [Self-published]. < www.brainsave.com >

Elliott, C. (2016). *The ghost in my brain: How a concussion stole my life and how the new science of brain plasticity helped me get it back.* Viking Penguin.

Engel, D. (2017). *The concussion repair manual: A practical guide to recovering from traumatic brain injuries.* Lifestyle Entrepreneurs Press.

King, N. S. (2015). *Overcoming mild traumatic brain injury and post-concussion symptoms: A self-help guide using evidence-based techniques.* Robinson.

Mason, D. J. (2004). *The mild traumatic brain injury workbook: Your program for regaining cognitive function and overcoming emotional pain.* New Harbinger Publications.

Nedd, K. J. (2020). *Concussion: Traumatic brain injury from head to tail.* Archway Publishing.

Steadman, S. (Ed.), & Zellmer, A. (Ed.) (2021). *Concussion discussions: A functional approach to recovery after brain injury.* Faces of TBI.

Wand, P. H. (2019). *The concussion cure: 3 proven methods to heal your brain.* [Self-published].

Zellmer A. (Ed.). *The Brain Health Magazine.* < www.thebrainhealthmagazine.com >

Concussion Recovery Online Courses

Concussion Compass. *Concussion compass.* < www.concussioncompass.com >

Complete Concussion Management. *The concussion fix.* < www.concussiondoc.io/courses/the-concussion-fix/ >

Chapek, K. *Concussion recovery program.* < www.amenuniversity.com/au-concussion-rescue >

Wienhoven, M. *Cure my concussion course*. < www.lifeyana.com/courses/
cure-my-concussion-course/ >
van de Ree, S. *The Concussion Community*. < www.theconcussioncommunity.
com/my-courses >

Concussion and Brain Injury Blogs

Balaster, C. *Adventures in brain injury*. < www.adventuresinbraininjury.com >
Website, blog and podcast of Cavin Balaster, severe brain injury
survivor and author of 'How to Feed a Brain'.
Cognitivefx. *The Cognitive FX blog*. < www.cognitivefxusa.com > A great
source of information on traumatic brain injury and concussions from
this world-class treatment centre in the USA.
Fallis, J. *Optimal living dynamics: Practical brain and mental health solutions*.
< www.optimallivingdynamics.com > Website and blog of Jordan
Fallis, concussion survivor and brain health coach.
Heisig, M. *Dr. Mark Heisig: Healthy on purpose*. <https://www.drheisig.com/
blog> Naturopathic doctor and concussion specialist. Dr. Heisig also
has a YouTube channel, Mark Heisig, ND.
Lewis, M. *Brain Health Education and Research Institute*.
< www.brainhealtheducation.org > A great source of information,
especially for the omega-3 protocol for brain injury recovery.
Marshall, C. *Complete Concussion Management*.
< http://www.completeconcussions.com/resources/ > Dr. Marshall
also has a YouTube channel, CompleteConcussionManagement and a
podcast, Ask Concussion Doc.
Munt, M. *Jumbled brain blog*. < www.jumbledbrain.com/blog/ > Website
and blog of Michelle Munt, traumatic brain injury survivor.
Nedd, K. J. *Concussion/TBI blog*. < www.concussiontbi.com/blog > Blog
and website of Dr Kester J. Nedd, Concussion and TBI specialist and
neurologist at Design Neuroscience Center.
Sequoia, C. *The Foggy Shore*. < www.thefoggyshore.wordpress.com/ > Blog
by someone recovering from concussion.
Wienhoven, M. *The post-concussion syndrome blog*. < www.lifeyana.com/
blog/ > Blog of Melanie Wienhoven, concussion survivor. Melanie also
has a YouTube channel, Lifeyana.
Zellmer, A. *Faces of TBI blog*. < www.facesoftbi.com/blog/ > Blog and
podcast of Amy Zellmer, concussion survivor. Amy also has a YouTube
channel, TBI TV, featuring interviews with concussion experts.

Concussion and Brain Injury Organizations

In the UK

Brain and Spine Foundation: < www.brainandspine.org >
Brain Injury Group: < www.braininjurygroup.co.uk >
Child Brain Injury Trust: < www.childbraininjurytrust.co.uk >
Headway: < www.headway.org.uk > Helpline: 0808 800 2244
PoTS (Postural Tachycardia Syndrome) UK: < www.potsuk.org >
Samaritans: < www.samaritans.org > Free 24/7 phone crisis helpline: 116 123
Same You: < www.sameyou.org/recovery_at_home >
Shout: < www.giveusashout.org > Free 24/7 text crisis line: 85258
UKABIF (UK Acquired Brain Injury Forum) Lobby organization: < www.ukabif.org.uk >

International

Brain Line: < www.brainline.org >
Brain Injury Association of America: < www.biausa.org >
Brain Injury Association of Canada: < www.braininjurycanada.ca >
Concussion Alliance: < www.concussionalliance.org >
Concussion Legacy Foundation: < www.concussionlegacyfoundation.com >
Dysautonomia International: < www.dysautonomiainternational.org >
Global Brain Injury Awareness CIC: < www.globalbia.org >
Love Your Brain Foundation: < www.loveyourbrain.com >
Pink Concussions: Focuses on concussions in women: < www.pinkconcussions.com >
Power of Patients: < www.powerofpatients.com >

Exercise

APPI (Australian Physiotherapy and Pilates Institute). Pilates classes, available on monthly subscription. < www.appi.tv >
Peter Appel. Movingness exercise programme. < www.movingness.com >
UBMD Orthopaedics and Sports Medicine. The Buffalo Concussion Treadmill Test (BCTT). < www.ubortho.com/services/concussion-management-center/ >
Kseny Grey. Qigong with Kseny. YouTube. < www.youtube.com/c/QigongwithKseny >
Lee Holden. Qigong exercises. YouTube. < www.youtube.com/c/HoldenQigong >
Emily Lark. Back to Life System to relieve back pain. < www.backpainstretch.com >

Love Your Brain. Yoga for people with brain injuries.
< www.loveyourbrain.com >

Shriya Maharaj. Propel Physiotherapy has a few free gentle exercise videos for people recovering from brain injury. < www.propelphysiotherapy. com/author/shriya-maharaj >

Svelte One & Done. 7-minute sprint interval training (SIT) exercise programme. < https://go.riseworkouts.com/ >

Lucy Wyndham-Read. Lots of short and longer exercise routines for all abilities, including some for people with disabilities and injuries. YouTube. < www.youtube.com/user/LWRFitnessChannel >

Nervous System and Trauma

Bashir, K. (2011). *Dizzyclear: Understanding dizziness and vertigo, their management and home treatments.* Grosvenor House Publishing.

Berceli, D. Trauma release exercises (TRE). < www.traumaprevention.com >

Dana, D. (2020, June 16). *Deb Dana: Befriending your nervous system.* [Audio podcast] < https://resources.soundstrue.com/podcast/deb-dana-befriending-your-nervous-system/ >

Dana, D. (2020). *Polyvagal exercises for safety and connection: 50 client-centred practices.* W. W. Norton & Company.

Dana, D. *Deb Dana's rhythm of regulation: The science of feeling safe enough to fall in love with life and take the risks of living.* < www.rhythmofregulation.com >

Levine, P. (2010). *In an unspoken voice: How the body releases trauma and restores goodness.* North Atlantic Books.

Irene Lyon – nervous system expert. Website: < www.irenelyon.com > and YouTube channel: < www.youtube.com/c/IreneLyon >

Porges, S. (2017). *The pocket guide to the polyvagal theory: The transformative power of feeling safe.* W. W. Norton & Company.

Rosenberg, S. (2017). *Accessing the healing power of the vagus nerve: Self-help exercises for anxiety, depression, trauma and autism.* North Atlantic Books.

Scaer, R. (2005). *The trauma spectrum: Hidden wounds and human resiliency.* W. W. Norton & Company.

Scaer, R. (2014). *The body bears the burden: Trauma, dissociation, and disease.* Routledge.

van der Kolk, B. (2015). *The body keeps the score: Mind, brain and body in the transformation of trauma.* Viking.

Neuroplasticity, Brain Health and Stress Management

Bolte Taylor, J. (2021). *Whole brain living: The anatomy of choice and the four characters that drive our life.* Hay House Inc.

Breuning, L. G. (2016). *Habits of a happy brain: Retrain your brain to boost your serotonin, dopamine, oxytocin and endorphin levels.* Adams Media.

Byron, K. *The work of Byron Katie.* < www.thework.com. >

Chatterjee, R. (2018). *The stress solution: The 4 steps to a calmer, happier, healthier you.* Penguin.

Chopra, D., & Tanzi, R. (2012). *Super brain: Unleashing the explosive power of your mind to maximize health, happiness and spiritual well-being.* Harmony.

Doidge, N. (2008). *The brain that changes itself: Stories of personal triumph from the frontiers of brain science.* Viking.

Doidge, N. (2016). *The brain's way of healing: Stories of remarkable recoveries and discoveries.* Penguin Life.

Fletcher, E. (2019). *Stress less, accomplish more: The 15-minute meditation programme for extraordinary performance.* Bluebird.

Hickmott, O. (2009). *Recover your energy and end fatigue by using energy enhanced NLP and the power of your mind.* MX Publishing.

Kwik, J. (2020). *Limitless: Upgrade your brain, learn anything faster and unlock your exceptional life.* Hay House Inc.

Leaf, C. (2021). *Cleaning up your mental mess: 5 simple scientifically proven steps to reduce, anxiety, stress and toxic thinking.* Baker Books.

Perlmutter, D. (2020). *Brain wash: Detox your mind for clearer thinking, deeper relationships and lasting happiness.* Little, Brown Spark.

The Minded Institute. *Yoga Therapy London: Yoga & mindfulness programmes in London & the UK.* < www.themindedinstitute.com >

Whitten, A. (2018.) *The ultimate guide to red light therapy: How to use red and near-infrared light therapy for anti-aging, fat loss, muscle gain, performance enhancement, and brain optimization.* [Self-published].

Apps

Calm: < www.calm.com >

Headspace: < www.headspace.com/headspace-meditation-app >

Neumind. *Alfred, for ABI rehabilitation.* [App, currently in beta]. Available via the Apple App Store or Google Play Store.

Nutrition and Supplements

I (Anna) buy most of my supplements from:
Nature's Best: www.naturesbest.co.uk
Ocean's Alive: www.oceansalive.co.uk
Oxford Vitality: www.oxfordvitality.co.uk

General Information about Nutrition and Supplements

Axe, J., Bollinger, T., & Rubin, J. (2016). *Essential oils: Ancient medicine.* Axe Wellness LLC.

Axe J. *Dr Axe: Health and fitness news, recipes, natural remedies.* < www.draxe.com >

Balaster, C. (2018). *How to feed a brain: Nutrition for optimal brain function and repair.* Feed A Brain LLC.

Healthline Media. *Healthline: Medical information and health advice you can trust.* < www.healthline.com >

Kelly, R., & Mackintosh, A. (2016). *The happy kitchen: Good mood food.* Simon & Schuster Australia.

Kharazzian, D. (2013). *Why isn't my brain working?: A revolutionary understanding of brain decline and effective strategies to recover your brain's health.* Elephant Press.

Lambert, R. (2017). *Re-nourish: A simple way to eat well.* Yellow Kite.

Lewis, M. D. (2016). *When brains collide: What every athlete and parent should know about the prevention and treatment of concussions and head injuries.* [Self-published].

Myers, A. (2018). *The Autoimmune solution cookbook.* HarperOne.

Prasad, K. N. (2016). *Treat concussion, TBI and PTSD with vitamins & antioxidants.* Healing Arts Press.

Sherzai, D., & Sherzai, A. (2021). *The 30-day Alzheimer's solution: The definitive food and lifestyle guide to preventing cognitive decline.* HarperOne.

Sullivan, T. (2012). *Nourish your noggin: Brain-building foods and easy-to-make recipes to hasten your healing from mild traumatic brain injury (concussion and post concussion syndrome).* Outskirts Press Inc.

Wahls, T. (2017). *The Wahls protocol: A radical new way to treat all chronic autoimmune conditions using paleo principles.* Avery.

Pain

Curable: A different approach to your pain. [App]. < www.curablehealth.com >

Gauci, M., & Clarke, D. *Path to pain free: The 25 day program to overcome mindbody chronic pain, and pave your way to a more fulfilling life.* < https://www.painoutsidethebox.com/path-to-pain-free >

Kuttner, J. (2017). *Life after pain: Break free of chronic pain and get your life back.* [Self-published]. < www.lifeafterpain.com >

Schubiner, H. (2016). *Unlearn your pain: A 28-day process to reprogram your brain.* < www.unlearnyourpain.com/unlearn-your-pain-book/ >

Sizer, P. (2019). *Chronic pain the drug-free way.* Sheldon Press.

Stress Illness Recovery Practitioners' Association (SIRPA). *SIRPA UK.* < www.sirpa.org >

Vestibular migraine: Understanding the condition, symptoms & treatments. < www.vestibularmigraine.co.uk >

Recovering from a Car Accident

McKay, D. (2021). *Talk crash to me: What to expect after surviving a motor vehicle collision and how to manage your recovery.* [Self-published].

Poole Heller, D., & Heller, L. S. (2001). *Crash course: A self-healing guide to auto accident trauma and recovery.* North Atlantic Books.

Zender, J. (2021). *Recovering from your car accident: The complete guide to reclaiming your life.* Rowman & Littlefield.

Therapy

Hayes, S. C., & Smith, S. (2005). *Get out of your mind and into your life: The new acceptance and commitment therapy.* New Harbinger Publications.

McAdam, E. *Therapy in a nutshell.* YouTube. < www.youtube.com/c/TherapyinaNutshell >

Smith, J. (2022). *Why has nobody told me this before?* HarperCollins.

Train Your Brain

Designs for Strong Minds. *Paper and pencil brain games.* < www.designsforstrongminds.com/paper-exercises >

Designs for Strong Minds. *Digital brain games.* [Apps.] < www.designsforstrongminds.com/mobile-apps#tbipap >

Jim Kwik. *Jim Kwik: Courses.* < www.jimkwik.com/courses>

Levi, J. *Become A Speed Demon 2: Productivity hacks to have more time.* < www.udemy.com >

Levi, J. *Become A Super Learner 2: Learn speed reading and boost memory.*
< www.udemy.com >
Lumosity. *Lumosity brain training: Challenge & improve your mind.* [App]
< www.lumosity.com >
Marisk, S. *Neuroplasticity masterclass: Unleash the power of your brain.*
< www.udemy.com >

Products

Body Back Buddy: trigger point therapy: < www.bodyback.com >
C-Rod: diagnose concussion and treat potential associated vision
problems. < www.concussionrecovery.net >
The Dyslexia Shop: coloured overlays for reading text.
< www.thedyslexiashop.co.uk >
Flare Audio: earplugs (try the Calmer, Isolate or Sleeep earplugs).
< www.flareaudio.com >
f.lux: a free blue light filter for screens. < www.justgetflux.com >
Happy Eye: glasses with coloured lenses. < www.happyeye.co.uk >
Tisserand: sleep spray and essential oils. < www.tisserand.com >

Index